Implementation and Scale Up of Point of Care (POC) Diagnostics in ResourceLimited Settings

Implementation and Scale Up of Point of Care (POC) Diagnostics in ResourceLimited Settings

Editors

Tivani Mashamba-Thompson
Paul K. Drain

MDPI • Basel • Beijing • Wuhan • Barcelona • Belgrade • Manchester • Tokyo • Cluj • Tianjin

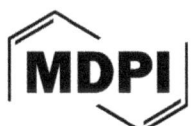

Editors
Tivani Mashamba-Thompson
University of Limpopo
South Africa

Paul K. Drain
University of Washington
USA

Editorial Office
MDPI
St. Alban-Anlage 66
4052 Basel, Switzerland

This is a reprint of articles from the Special Issue published online in the open access journal *Diagnostics* (ISSN 2075-4418) (available at: https://www.mdpi.com/journal/diagnostics/special_issues/poc_diagnostics).

For citation purposes, cite each article independently as indicated on the article page online and as indicated below:

LastName, A.A.; LastName, B.B.; LastName, C.C. Article Title. *Journal Name* **Year**, *Article Number*, Page Range.

ISBN 978-3-03943-170-0 (Hbk)
ISBN 978-3-03943-171-7 (PDF)

© 2020 by the authors. Articles in this book are Open Access and distributed under the Creative Commons Attribution (CC BY) license, which allows users to download, copy and build upon published articles, as long as the author and publisher are properly credited, which ensures maximum dissemination and a wider impact of our publications.

The book as a whole is distributed by MDPI under the terms and conditions of the Creative Commons license CC BY-NC-ND.

Contents

About the Editors vii

Tivani P. Mashamba-Thompson and Paul K. Drain
Point-of-Care Diagnostic Services as an Integral Part of Health Services during the Novel Coronavirus 2019 Era
Reprinted from: *Diagnostics* **2020**, *10*, 449, doi:10.3390/diagnostics10070449 . . . . **1**

Shabashini Reddy, Andrew Gibbs, Elizabeth Spooner, Noluthando Ngomane, Tarylee Reddy, Nozipho —Luthuli, Gita Ramjee, Anna Coutsoudis and Photini Kiepiela
Assessment of the Impact of Rapid Point-of-Care CD4 Testing in Primary Healthcare Clinic Settings: A Survey Study of Client and Provider Perspectives
Reprinted from: *Diagnostics* **2020**, *10*, 81, doi:10.3390/diagnostics10020081 . . . . **5**

Tivani P. Mashamba-Thompson, Paul K. Drain, Desmond Kuupiel and Benn Sartorius
Impact of Implementing Antenatal Syphilis Point-of-Care Testing on Maternal Mortality in KwaZulu-Natal, South Africa: An Interrupted Time Series Analysis
Reprinted from: *Diagnostics* **2019**, *9*, 218, doi:10.3390/diagnostics9040218 . . . . **23**

Desmond Kuupiel, Kwame M. Adu, Vitalis Bawontuo, Duncan A. Adogboba, Paul K. Drain, Mosa Moshabela and Tivani P. Mashamba-Thompson
Geographical Accessibility to Glucose-6-Phosphate Dioxygenase Deficiency Point-of-Care Testing for Antenatal Care in Ghana
Reprinted from: *Diagnostics* **2020**, *10*, 229, doi:10.3390/diagnostics10040229 . . . . **33**

Desmond Kuupiel, Kwame M. Adu, Vitalis Bawontuo, Duncan A. Adogboba and Tivani P. Mashamba-Thompson
Estimating the Spatial Accessibility to Blood Group and Rhesus Type Point-of-Care Testing for Maternal Healthcare in Ghana
Reprinted from: *Diagnostics* **2019**, *9*, 175, doi:10.3390/diagnostics9040175 . . . . **47**

Anna M. Maw, Brittany Galvin, Ricardo Henri, Micheal Yao, Bruno Exame, Michelle Fleshner, Meredith P. Fort and Megan A. Morris
Stakeholder Perceptions of Point-of-Care Ultrasound Implementation in Resource-Limited Settings
Reprinted from: *Diagnostics* **2019**, *9*, 153, doi:10.3390/diagnostics9040153 . . . . **61**

Davinder Ramsingh, Michael Ma, Danny Quy Le, Warren Davis, Mark Ringer, Briahnna Austin and Cameron Ricks
Feasibility Evaluation of Commercially Available Video Conferencing Devices to Technically Direct Untrained Nonmedical Personnel to Perform a Rapid Trauma Ultrasound Examination
Reprinted from: *Diagnostics* **2019**, *9*, 188, doi:10.3390/diagnostics9040188 . . . . **73**

Nkosinothando Chamane, Desmond Kuupiel and Tivani Phosa Mashamba-Thompson
Stakeholders' Perspectives for the Development of a Point-of-Care Diagnostics Curriculum in Rural Primary Clinics in South Africa—Nominal Group Technique
Reprinted from: *Diagnostics* **2020**, *10*, 195, doi:10.3390/diagnostics10040195 . . . . **83**

Tafadzwa Dzinamarira, Collins Kamanzi and Tivani Phosa Mashamba-Thompson
Key Stakeholders' Perspectives on Implementation and Scale up of HIV Self-Testing in Rwanda
Reprinted from: *Diagnostics* **2020**, *10*, 194, doi:10.3390/diagnostics10040194 . . . . **95**

Davinder Ramsingh, Cori Van Gorkom, Matthew Holsclaw, Scott Nelson, Martin De La Huerta, Julian Hinson and Emilie Selleck
Use of a Smartphone-Based Augmented Reality Video Conference App to Remotely Guide a Point of Care Ultrasound Examination
Reprinted from: *Diagnostics* **2019**, *9*, 159, doi:10.3390/diagnostics9040159 . . . . **107**

Tivani P. Mashamba-Thompson and Ellen Debra Crayton
Blockchain and Artificial Intelligence Technology for Novel Coronavirus Disease 2019 Self-Testing
Reprinted from: *Diagnostics* **2020**, *10*, 198, doi:10.3390/diagnostics10040198 . . . . **113**

Thokozani Khubone, Boikhutso Tlou and Tivani Phosa Mashamba-Thompson
Electronic Health Information Systems to Improve Disease Diagnosis and Management at Point-of-Care in Low and Middle Income Countries: A Narrative Review
Reprinted from: *Diagnostics* **2020**, *10*, 327, doi:10.3390/diagnostics10050327 . . . . **117**

G-Young Van, Adeola Onasanya, Jo van Engelen, Oladimeji Oladepo and Jan Carel Diehl
Improving Access to Diagnostics for Schistosomiasis Case Management in Oyo State, Nigeria: Barriers and Opportunities
Reprinted from: *Diagnostics* **2020**, *10*, 328, doi:10.3390/diagnostics10050328 . . . . **127**

About the Editors

Tivani Mashamba-Thompson is a full professor in the Faculty of Health Sciences, University of Limpopo, South Africa. She is a medical scientist (Molecular Biology), and is registered with the Health Profession Council South Africa. Mashamba-Thompson conducts research on the implementation of point-of-care diagnostics for the underserved population in resource-limited settings, and performs evaluation studies for new point-of-care diagnostics in these settings. She completed her Honors Degree in Applied Biomedical Science at the University of Surrey, UK, and her master's in Pharmaceutical Science (summa cum laude) and PhD in Public Health at the University of KwaZulu-Natal. Her postdoctoral training was completed with the Canadian HIV Clinical Research Network. At the University of Limpopo, Mashamba-Thompson coordinates and teaches research methods and program evaluation modules to Masters students in the Department of Public Health. She also serves as a research chairperson for the Department of Public Health, and is a member of the university senior management committee. Prior to joining the University of Limpopo, Tivani was an academic leader and research and associate professor at the University of KwaZulu-Natal. She is the author of more than 80 peer-reviewed articles in accredited journals, including high impact journals, such as Lancet and Nature. To date, she has led and supersized five funded research projects, and supervised 14 master's students and two PhD students to completion. Tivani is a member of the COVID-19 scientific advisory committee for the Limpopo Province, and she is one of the site primary investigators for a national study aimed at the community-based validation of new COVID-19 point-of-care tests in South Africa. Prof. Mashamba-Thompson's research work on point-of-care diagnostics has been recognized nationally and internationally. She achieved her first NRF (National Research Framework) rating in 2017, and she was invited to join the University College London (UCL) Collaboration for the Advancement of Sustainable Medical Innovation (CASMI) fellowship. Mashamba-Thompson is also a Harvard Medical School (HMS) alumna; she completed the HMS 2017/2018 Global Clinical Scholars Research Training (GCSRT) with commendation.

Paul K. Drain, MD, MPH, is an assistant professor in the Departments of Global Health, Medicine (Infectious Diseases), and Epidemiology at the University of Washington, and a practicing Infectious Disease physician at Harborview Medical Center and the University of Washington Medical Center in Seattle. His research group focuses on the development, evaluation and implementation of diagnostic testing and clinic-based screening, including novel point-of-care technologies, to improve clinical care and patient-centered outcomes for tuberculosis and HIV in resource-limited settings. He is Associate Director of the Tuberculosis Research and Training Center at the University of Washington. He research has been supported by several institutes of the National Institutes of Health, the Infectious Disease Society of America, the Bill and Melinda Gates Foundation, Harvard Global Health Institute, both the UW's and Harvard's Center for AIDS Research, and the AIDS Healthcare Foundation. He has authored several global health books and received awards from the Infectious Disease Society of America, and a Faculty Teaching Award from Harvard Medical School.

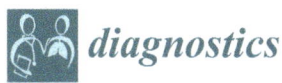

Editorial

Point-of-Care Diagnostic Services as an Integral Part of Health Services during the Novel Coronavirus 2019 Era

Tivani P. Mashamba-Thompson [1],* and Paul K. Drain [2,3,4,5]

1. Department of Public Health, University of Limpopo, Polokwane, Limpopo Province 0727, South Africa
2. International Clinical Research Center, Department of Global Health, University of Washington, Seattle, WA 98195-7965, USA; pkdrain@uw.edu
3. Division of Infectious Diseases, Department of Medicine, University of Washington, Seattle, WA 98195-7965, USA
4. Department of Epidemiology, University of Washington, Seattle, WA 98195-7965, USA
5. Department of Surgery, Harvard University, Massachusetts General Hospital, Boston, MA 02114, USA
* Correspondence: tivani.mashamba@ul.ac.za

Received: 2 July 2020; Accepted: 2 July 2020; Published: 3 July 2020

Abstract: Point-of-care (POC) diagnostic services are commonly associated with pathology laboratory services. This issue presents a holistic approach to POC diagnostics services from a variety of disciplines including pathology, radiological and information technology as well as mobile technology and artificial intelligence. This highlights the need for transdisciplinary collaboration to ensure the efficient development and implementation of point-of-care diagnostics. The advent of the novel coronavirus 2019 (COVID-19) pandemic has prompted rapid advances in the development of new POC diagnostics. Global private and public sector agencies have significantly increased their investment in the development of POC diagnostics. There is no longer a question about the availability and accessibility of POC diagnostics. The question is "how can POC diagnostic services be integrated into health services in way that is useful and acceptable in the COVID-19 era?".

Keywords: point-of-care diagnostics; healthcare services; COVID-19 era

---

Point-of-care (POC) refers to the location where healthcare interventions are carried out. These interventions can be carried out in a variety of settings including in the home, in the office, in the community and at a healthcare facility. Disease diagnosis or testing is one of the healthcare interventions that can be carried at POC and referred to as POC diagnostic services or POC testing. POC testing is performed using various POC diagnostics to enable the near-patient detection and monitoring of disease conditions in order to inform prognoses, guide treatment choices and predict treatment responses [1]. The advent of POC diagnostics in resource-limited settings has enhanced diagnostic capacity and helped to improve access to healthcare in areas where disease burden is high and diagnosis remains a weak point in the healthcare system [2–4]. The most commonly used and accessible POC diagnostics in most of these settings are pathology tests such as HIV and malaria tests [5,6]. This issue has demonstrated the use of pathology, radiological and information technology systems as well as mobile technology and artificial intelligence for POC diagnostic services. The advent of the novel coronavirus 2019 (COVID-19) pandemic has put POC diagnostics in the spotlight and prompted rapid advances in the development of POC diagnostics and their delivery approaches. Global private and public sector agencies have significantly increased their investment in the development of POC diagnostics. There is no longer a question about the availability, accessibility and acceptability of point-of-care diagnostics services. The question is "how can point-of-care diagnostics services be integrated into current health services in way that is useful and acceptable in the COVID-19 era?".

This issue presents translational research presenting evidence of the benefits of implementing POC diagnostics and strategies to help integrate POC diagnostic services into current healthcare services.

The development of new evidence-based POC diagnostics and the replication of these diagnostics to extend their reach is a global health priority. The appropriate integration of new POC diagnostics approaches is crucial for ensuring desirable outcomes. The implementation of POC healthcare interventions such as POC testing ought to be relevant to each specific context and sensitive to local culture. Factors such as infrastructure, resources, values and the characteristics of the participants can influence the implementation, scalability and sustainability of health interventions. A study conducted in Nigeria calls for community education, screening for schistosomiasis, and the enhancement of diagnostic capacity and strengthening of the capability of health workers through point-of-care diagnostics [2]. Our previous research demonstrates the need for improving the accessibility of Glucose-6-Phosphate Dioxygenase Deficiency [7] and blood-group and rhesus-type tests [8] as part of antenatal care services in malaria regions. These studies also highlight the need to update the World Health Organization (WHO) essential diagnostics (EDL) and for the development of content specific for POC diagnostics lists during the COVID-19 era. Following the implementation of recommended diagnostics at the POC, there is a need for optimizing the development of POC diagnostics delivery approaches to ensure continual quality service delivery, particularly among underserved populations and resource-limited settings.

Research suggests the need for training healthcare workers to improve POC diagnostic service delivery in resource-limited settings [9–11]. Primary Healthcare (PHC) healthcare workers in rural South Africa suggested an experiential learning approach using eLearning to help them maintain their competence in terms of HIV POC diagnostics service delivery [12]. Despite the wide availability of PHC-based HIV testing services, there are still substantial gaps. Access to these services is a challenge to key populations such as men in sub-Saharan Africa. A study conducted in Rwanda focusing on optimizing the implementation and scale up of HIV self-testing approaches for HIV to help improve men's engagement with HIV services has identified the following priority areas: the creation of awareness; the training those involved in the implementation process; the regulation of the selling of the self-test kits; the reduction of the costs of acquiring the self-test kits through the provision of subsidies; and ensuring the consistent availability of the self-test kits were identified [13]. Previous research shows that the advancement of mobile technology and improved data affordability has benefited the successful implementation of POC diagnostics approaches such as self-testing [14]. Smartphone technology and POC ultrasound (POCUS) devices have proven to be key examples of how technological advances are poised to improve healthcare delivery in resource-limited settings [11,15]. POC diagnostics has the potential help with the much-needed rapid development of information systems within the health sector through artificial intelligence and machine learning-linked POC diagnostics [16]. The integration of POC diagnostics with existing Health Information Systems should help to improve disease diagnostics and management [17].

The integration of available POC diagnostics into our current healthcare service needs to be prioritized to aid the prevention and management of current pandemics and in preparation for future pandemics. It is clear that the successful implementation of point-of-care diagnostics requires a transdisciplinary approach. Investment in transdisciplinary research platforms for POC diagnostics is recommended. These platforms can also foster improved awareness and recognition of POC diagnostics services as a standalone healthcare service and development of POC diagnostics curricula for the training of a new cadre of healthcare workers, dedicated to POC diagnostic services. The successful implementation of such platforms requires multidisciplinary and multi-sectorial stakeholder involvement including higher education institutions, diagnostics and information and mobile technology developers and providers as well as implementers and users of POC diagnostic services.

Funding: This research received no external funding.

Conflicts of Interest: The authors declare no conflict of interest.

References

1. Billings, P.R. Three barriers to innovative diagnostics. *Nat. Biotechnol.* **2006**, *24*, 917–918. [CrossRef] [PubMed]
2. Van, G.-Y.; Onasanya, A.; Van Engelen, J.; Oladepo, O.; Diehl, J.C. Improving Access to Diagnostics for Schistosomiasis Case Management in Oyo State, Nigeria: Barriers and Opportunities. *Diagnostics* **2020**, *10*, 328. [CrossRef] [PubMed]
3. Reddy, S.; Gibbs, A.; Spooner, E.; Ngomane, N.; Reddy, T.; Nozipho Luthuli Ramjee, G.; Coutsoudis, A. Assessment of the Impact of Rapid Point-of-Care CD4 Testing in Primary Healthcare Clinic Settings: A Survey Study of Client and Provider Perspectives. *Diagnostics* **2020**, *10*, 81. [CrossRef] [PubMed]
4. Mashamba-Thompson, T.P.; Drain, P.K.; Kuupiel, D.; Sartorius, B. Impact of Implementing Antenatal Syphilis Point-of-Care Testing on Maternal Mortality in KwaZulu-Natal, South Africa: An Interrupted Time Series Analysis. *Diagnostics* **2019**, *9*, 218. [CrossRef] [PubMed]
5. Mashamba-Thompson, T.P.; Sartorius, B.; Drain, P.K. Operational assessment of point-of-care diagnostics in rural primary healthcare clinics of KwaZulu-Natal, South Africa: a cross-sectional survey. *BMC Health Serv. Res.* **2018**, *18*, 380. [CrossRef] [PubMed]
6. Kuupiel, D.; Tlou, B.; Bawontuo, V.; Mashamba-Thompson, T.P. Accessibility of Point-of-Care Diagnostic Services for Maternal Health in Lower Healthcare Facilities in Northern Ghana: A Cross-Sectional Survey. *SSRN Electron. J.* **2018**. [CrossRef]
7. Kuupiel, D.; Adu, K.M.; Bawontuo, V.; Adogboba, D.A.; Drain, P.K.; Moshabela, M.; Mashamba-Thompson, T.P. Geographical Accessibility to Glucose-6-Phosphate Dioxygenase Deficiency Point-of-Care Testing for Antenatal Care in Ghana. *Diagnostics* **2020**, *10*, 229. [CrossRef] [PubMed]
8. Kuupiel, D.; Adu, K.M.; Bawontuo, V.; Adogboba, D.A.; Mashamba-Thompson, T.P. Estimating the Spatial Accessibility to Blood Group and Rhesus Type Point-of-Care Testing for Maternal Healthcare in Ghana. *Diagnostics* **2019**, *9*, 175. [CrossRef] [PubMed]
9. Maw, A.M.; Galvin, B.; Henri, R.; Yao, M.; Exame, B.; Fleshner, M.; Fort, M.P.; Morris, M.A.; Yao, M.S. Stakeholder Perceptions of Point-of-Care Ultrasound Implementation in Resource-Limited Settings. *Diagnostics* **2019**, *9*, 153. [CrossRef] [PubMed]
10. Mashamba-Thompson, T.P.; Jama, N.A.; Sartorius, B.; Drain, P.K.; Thompson, R.M. Implementation of Point-of-Care Diagnostics in Rural Primary Healthcare Clinics in South Africa: Perspectives of Key Stakeholders. *Diagnostics* **2017**, *7*, 3. [CrossRef] [PubMed]
11. Ramsingh, D.; Ma, M.; Le, D.Q.; Davis, W.; Ringer, M.; Austin, B.; Ricks, C. Feasibility Evaluation of Commercially Available Video Conferencing Devices to Technically Direct Untrained Nonmedical Personnel to Perform a Rapid Trauma Ultrasound Examination. *Diagnostics* **2019**, *9*, 188. [CrossRef] [PubMed]
12. Chamane, N.; Kuupiel, D.; Mashamba-Thompson, T.P. Stakeholders' Perspectives for the Development of a Point-of-Care Diagnostics Curriculum in Rural Primary Clinics in South Africa—Nominal Group Technique. *Diagnostics* **2020**, *10*, 195. [CrossRef] [PubMed]
13. Dzinamarira, T.; Kamanzi, C.; Mashamba-Thompson, T.P. Key Stakeholders' Perspectives on Implementation and Scale up of HIV Self-Testing in Rwanda. *Diagnostics* **2020**, *10*, 194. [CrossRef] [PubMed]
14. Wood, C.; Thomas, M.R.; Budd, J.; Mashamba-Thompson, T.P.; Herbst, K.; Pillay, D.; Peeling, R.W.; Johnson, A.M.; McKendry, R.A.; Stevens, M.M. Taking connected mobile-health diagnostics of infectious diseases to the field. *Nature* **2019**, *566*, 467–474. [CrossRef] [PubMed]
15. Ramsingh, D.; Van Gorkom, C.; Holsclaw, M.; Nelson, S.; De La Huerta, M.; Hinson, J.; Selleck, E. Use of a Smartphone-Based Augmented Reality Video Conference App to Remotely Guide a Point of Care Ultrasound Examination. *Diagnostics* **2019**, *9*, 159. [CrossRef] [PubMed]
16. Mashamba-Thompson, T.P.; Crayton, E.D. Blockchain and Artificial Intelligence Technology for Novel Coronavirus Disease 2019 Self-Testing. *Diagnostics* **2020**, *10*, 198. [CrossRef] [PubMed]
17. Khubone, T.; Tlou, B.; Mashamba-Thompson, T.P. Electronic Health Information Systems to Improve Disease Diagnosis and Management at Point-of-Care in Low and Middle Income Countries: A Narrative Review. *Diagnostics* **2020**, *10*, 327. [CrossRef] [PubMed]

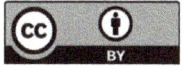

© 2020 by the authors. Licensee MDPI, Basel, Switzerland. This article is an open access article distributed under the terms and conditions of the Creative Commons Attribution (CC BY) license (http://creativecommons.org/licenses/by/4.0/).

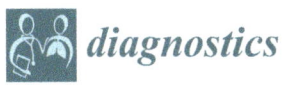

Article

Assessment of the Impact of Rapid Point-of-Care CD4 Testing in Primary Healthcare Clinic Settings: A Survey Study of Client and Provider Perspectives

Shabashini Reddy [1,2], Andrew Gibbs [3], Elizabeth Spooner [4], Noluthando Ngomane [5], Tarylee Reddy [6], Nozipho |Luthuli [7], Gita Ramjee [4], Anna Coutsoudis [8] and Photini Kiepiela [1,2,*]

1 South African Medical Research Council, Durban 4000, South Africa; Shabashini.reddy@mrc.ac.za
2 Wits Health Consortium, Parktown, Johannesburg 2091, South Africa
3 South African Medical Research Council, Gender and Health Research Unit, Durban Centre for Rural Health, University of KwaZulu Natal, Durban 4000, South Africa; Andrew.gibbs@mrc.ac.za
4 South African Medical Research Council, HIV Prevention Research Unit, Durban 3600, South Africa; Elizabeth.spooner@mrc.ac.za (E.S.); Gita.ramjee@mrc.ac.za (G.R.)
5 Occupational Health, Hillcrest, Durban 3610, South Africa; thando.frd.ngomane@gmail.com
6 South African Medical Research Council, Biostatistics Unit, Durban 4000, South Africa; Tarylee.reddy@mrc.ac.za
7 eThekwini Health Unit, Durban 4000, South Africa; Nozipho.Luthuli@durban.gov.za
8 School of Clinical Medicine, University of KwaZulu Natal, Durban 4000, South Africa; coutsoud@ukzn.ac.za
* Correspondence: kiepiela@gmail.com

Received: 5 November 2019; Accepted: 7 December 2019; Published: 1 February 2020

Abstract: Background: The high burden of disease in South Africa presents challenges to public health services. Point-of-care (POC) technologies have the potential to address these gaps and improve healthcare systems. This study ascertained the acceptability and impact of POC CD4 testing on patients' health and clinical management. Methods: We conducted a qualitative survey study with patients ($n = 642$) and healthcare providers ($n = 13$) at the Lancers Road (experienced POC) and Chesterville (non-experienced POC) primary healthcare (PHC) clinics from September 2015 to June 2016. Results: Patients (99%) at Lancers and Chesterville PHCs were positive about POC CD4 testing, identifying benefits: No loss/delay of test results (6.4%), cost/time saving (19.5%), and no anxiety (5.1%), and 58.2% were ready to initiate treatment. Significantly more patients at Chesterville than Lancers Road PHC felt POC would provide rapid clinical decision making (64.7% vs. 48.1%; $p < 0.0001$) and better clinic accessibility (40.4% vs. 24.7%; $p < 0.0001$) respectively. Healthcare providers thought same-day CD4 results would impact: Clinical management (46.2%), patient readiness (46.2%), and adherence (23.0%), and would reduce follow-up visits (7.7%), while 38.5% were concerned that further tests and training (15.4%) were required before antiretroviral therapy (ART) initiation. Conclusion: The high acceptability of POC CD4 testing and the immediate health, structural, and clinical management benefits necessitates POC implementation studies.

Keywords: point-of-care CD4+ t testing; qualitative survey; acceptability; patients; healthcare providers; primary healthcare clinics

1. Introduction

South Africa has an estimated population of 58.78 million with 7.97 million living with Human Immunodeficiency Virus (HIV), of whom 20% are women of reproductive age (15–49 years) [1], while the highest HIV prevalence ((27%) is in the province of KwaZulu Natal [1]. In September 2016, South Africa [2] adopted the World Health Organization (WHO) recommendations of universal treatment to all adults living with HIV, regardless of CD4 count [3], resulting in more than 4.5 million people taking antiretroviral therapy (ART), making it the largest ART programme globally [4].

Conventional HIV treatment and care services provided at primary healthcare (PHC) clinics in the public service in South Africa are largely unable to cope with the volume of patients entering the system, resulting in delayed and missed opportunities for treatment and ultimately unacceptably high levels of morbidity and mortality [5].

Diagnostic CD4 testing performed by conventional flow cytometry is centralized and offsite, provided by the National Health Laboratory Service (NHLS), serving >80% of the population [6]. There are several drawbacks of conventional testing, both from the patient and laboratory perspective, viz:

- Risk of losing patients who may not return due to cost and distance; delays in diagnosis and treatment initiation;
- Patients who seek healthcare elsewhere become nontraceable, giving wrong addresses to clinics further away for eligibility resulting in unnecessary repeat testing and higher workloads in some PHC clinics [7];
- Incomplete or incorrect completion of request forms or labelling of test tubes;
- The rejection of sample quality (insufficient or clotted specimen);
- Specimen damage or loss through transport;
- Misplacing of printed laboratory results at the clinic [7,8].

Instituting point-of-care (POC) CD4 testing in PHC clinics with the availability of same day results has the potential to address a number of these challenges for both patients and the health system. Additionally, POC testing brings with it greater patient satisfaction and helps with the morale of healthcare providers doing away with the "frustration" associated with conventional testing [9]. Daneau et al. (2016) [10] stated that the only objection to finger stick POC CD4 testing was due to pain/soreness. Additionally, some patients may decline POC testing as they may not feel emotionally/psychologically ready to receive same-day results [11].

Implementation of POC studies has demonstrated the reduction of pretreatment loss to follow-up in Mozambique [12,13], acceleration of ART initiation, but not retention, in care at 12 months [14], and reducing the time to diagnosis of multidrug resistance tuberculosis (TB) in South Africa [15]. In simulated cohort models of HIV-infected adults and pregnant women, the provision of same-day CD4 results was shown to result in better clinical outcomes and cost savings over the long term (five years) [16,17]. Another study focusing on POC processes across multiple diseases found that other challenges and delays were created with respect to the continual interaction of patient and healthcare [7].

Barriers to POC implementation have also been documented [7,18] where it was shown that POC testing needs to be integrated efficiently into the clinical care pathways. Otherwise it can result in increasing waiting time [19] and length of clinic visit [7,19–21].

Several studies have assessed the acceptability of POC assays, such as CD4 testing [10] and the POC viral load (VL) early infant diagnosis (EID) [9] in patients, resulting in better clinical outcomes [22,23]. The weaknesses of prior qualitative research were the small sample size and self-selecting sample in a study [24] or a project recruiting a specific population within the PHC or a hospital [9,10]. The strength of our work offers an unbiased alternative perspective of the general patient population within the PHC who was willing to give consent when referred for phlebotomy. The other advantage is the comparison of two PHC clinics with differing POC testing experiences.

At the time of undertaking this qualitative survey study, several POC technologies (Alere PIMA^{TM} CD4, [25] TB LAMP [26], and EID [9]), were being evaluated at the Lancers Road PHC clinic. It was therefore an opportune time to explore the provision of same-day POC CD4 test result as patients could relate these results to their health. Although guidelines have changed and CD4 tests have been replaced with VL testing for treatment adherence, the data presented here remain relevant in understanding how nurses and patients interpret and make sense of POC in PHC settings. We therefore sought to assess the acceptability, understanding, and perceptions in both client and healthcare provider perspective on the usefulness and impact of rapid POC CD4 testing in a POC research "experienced" site (Lancers Road PHC) compared to a research "naïve" site (Chesterville PHC).

2. Materials and Methods

2.1. Study Design

This was a qualitative survey study determining the acceptability, understanding, and perceptions from the client and healthcare provider perspective of the impact of the provision of POC CD4 testing in a PHC clinic setting. A qualitative survey utilises open-ended questions (rather than closed yes/no or agree/disagree questions) and delivers this to a larger sample of participants than is typical in a qualitative study [27]. This allows for the assessment and quantification of a variety of opinions without providing a fixed set of opinions for responses.

2.2. Study Population

The study population consisted of a convenience sample of clients presenting at the Lancers Road and Chesterville PHC clinics under the eThekwini Health Unit from 25 September 2015 to 30 June 2016. Individuals (>18 years old) who were referred to the "blood room" for phlebotomy (both HIV-1 negative and HIV-1 positive) and were willing to provide informed consent were included in the study.

2.3. Study Setting

Lancers Road PHC clinic is a busy primary health clinic (PHC) facility under the eThekwini Health Unit, situated in the centre of the convergence of the taxi rank from all the outlying areas into the city of Durban. Chesterville PHC is situated within the Chesterville community, serving a population of 15,840 [28] and situated 13.0 km from the centre of Durban.

Lancers Road PHC was considered a POC research "experienced" site as different studies were being undertaken evaluating several POC tests including POC CD4, whereas Chesterville PHC was a research "naïve" site as far as POC testing was concerned.

2.4. PHC Clinic Procedures

Both PHCs offered all PHC services seeing 250–400 patients per day. This included HIV Counselling and Testing (HCT) for walk-in patients, with both clinics performing on average 600–700 HCT/month. Both PHC clinics provided basic education sessions every morning in the waiting room covering different topics:

Chronic care (diabetes; hypertension; cardiovascular diseases);
Antenatal (breastfeeding; pregnancy; immunisations for children);
Cancer (breast and ovarian);
HIV education.

The PHC clinic procedures with respect to HIV Counselling and Testing (HCT) are depicted in Figure 1.

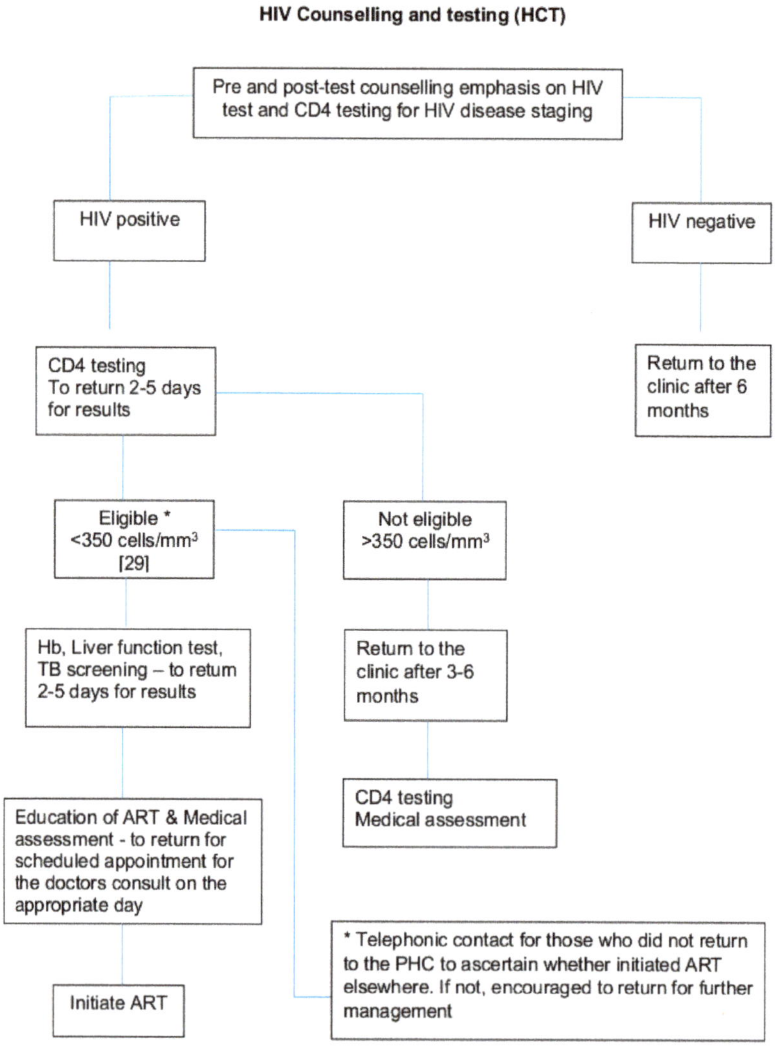

HIV Counselling and testing (HCT)

```
                    Pre and post-test counselling emphasis on HIV
                    test and CD4 testing for HIV disease staging

        HIV positive                                    HIV negative

        CD4 testing                                     Return to the
        To return 2-5 days                              clinic after 6
        for results                                     months

   Eligible *              Not eligible
   <350 cells/mm³          >350 cells/mm³
   [29]

   Hb, Liver function test,    Return to the
   TB screening – to return    clinic after 3-6
   2-5 days for results        months

                               CD4 testing
   Education of ART & Medical  Medical assessment
   assessment - to return for
   scheduled appointment for
   the doctors consult on the
   appropriate day

                               * Telephonic contact for those who did not return
                               to the PHC to ascertain whether initiated ART
                               elsewhere. If not, encouraged to return for further
        Initiate ART           management
```

Figure 1. Schematic flow of the PHC clinic procedures with respect to HIV Counselling and Testing (HCT) [29].

2.5. Study Procedures

Patients' requiring phlebotomy (both HIV-1 positive and HIV-1 negative) who were seen in the "blood room" by the counsellor/phlebotomist were approached by a study research assistant to participate in the study. Hence, there was no stigmatization for those that were HIV-1 infected as only the counsellor/phlebotomist and the patient knew what blood draw/s were required. They provided written informed consent, and then completed face-to-face questionnaires. If during enrollment patients asked what a POC test was, they were told, "It is a test you get back on the same day".

Patient questionnaires focused on their understanding and perceptions of a POC laboratory on-site providing same-day results, their interpretation of a CD4 test, and whether they were ready to start ART if eligible. For each question (5 in total), we initially asked participants a yes/no closed question. We specifically asked five questions:

1. Are you happy to receive a CD4 test result on the same day? ($n = 642$)
2. Would you rather wait for a CD4 test result or return to the clinic another day?
3. How long did it take to get your CD4 test result?
4. Do you know what a CD4 test result means?
5. Are you ready to start ART if eligible?

After each closed item, we asked a single open-ended question, probing their answer. Participants had three lines to answer on, however most just recorded short answers.

For healthcare providers, we approached all within the PHC and requested their participation. Questionnaires were also administered to the healthcare providers. Healthcare provider questionnaires mainly focused on their perception of the usefulness of same-day CD4 results to patients and their interpretation of the meaning of a CD4 test result, as well as the impact that same-day CD4 results would have on their workload, patient clinical management, and administration of ART initiation. Similarly, for each question (5 in total), we asked healthcare providers initially a yes/no closed question. We specifically asked 5 questions:

1. Do you think it is beneficial for the patient to get their CD4 result on the same day?
2. What was the impact on your workload in giving CD4 results to the patient on the same day?
3. Does having a CD4 result on the same day help you with patient management?
4. Do you know what a CD4 test result means?
5. Were you able to administer antiretrovirals (ARVs) to the patient on the same day you had the CD4 test result?

After each closed item, we asked a single open-ended question probing their answer. Nurses had 5 lines to answer on.

2.6. Data Handling and Recordkeeping

Study records were maintained safely in a locked cabinet on-site for the entire study period. The risks of participation were minimal. Confidentiality was maintained by assigning each patient/healthcare provider a unique study number and using the study number as the sole patient/healthcare provider identifier. Patient responses were entered into a specific database, which was secured using password-protected access systems.

2.7. Ethics

The study was approved by the Medical Research Council Research Ethics Committee (EC017-6/2015) as well as the eThekwini Research Ethics Committee (No. M.1/1/2 2 September 2015).

2.8. Statistical Considerations

2.8.1. Sample Size

The study was powered on patient acceptance of POC testing, which was assessed from the response to question 3.1 (Do you think it is a good idea to have a point of care laboratory in the clinic?). To detect a 90% POC test acceptance rate within a 7% margin of error at an alpha of 5%, 71 consenting patients were required. Assuming that 10% of HIV positive patients refused to consent to the study, approximately 80 HIV positive patients were required to reach the required sample size. Under the assumption that 25% of patients who were present for HIV testing were HIV positive, our sample size target was 320 patients in total at each PHC clinic, to be screened for entry into the study.

2.8.2. Statistical Analysis

The analysis of categorical outcomes is presented as frequencies and percentages.

As this was a qualitative survey study, data from the questionnaires from patients from each PHC clinic and healthcare provider (all nursing staff at the Lancers Road and Chesterville PHC clinics) were computed using coding. The binomial test with normal approximation was used to test whether proportions observed differed significantly between clinics. A 5% level of significance was used. Data were analyzed using Stata version 13.

To understand the variation qualitatively in people's responses, we did an open coding on participants' written answers to each question. We then organized the different small codes into larger themes, which connected codes together to understand the responses of participants. Once we had done this, we allocated each participant a response code and calculated the percentage and number who provided each reason for their answer.

3. Results

There were 642 patients interviewed, 322 at Lancers Road PHC and 320 at Chesterville PHC, of whom 272/322 (85%) and 233/320 (72.8%) were women with a median age of 32 and 34 years at Lancers Road and Chesterville PHC, respectively. No one refused to participate.

The overwhelming majority (99.5%) of patients in both the research "experienced" (Lancers Road; 322/322 (100%)) and "naïve" (Chesterville; 318/320 (99.4%)) PHC clinics welcomed the receipt of same-day CD4 test results ((a) in Table 1). Qualitatively, there were three reasons why patients were happy to receive their results immediately: Three-quarters (73.8%) said it was so they could receive medical care and help immediately, including starting ARVs if necessary. A fifth (19.5%) reported that it would save them time and money, as they would not need to return to the clinic. Meanwhile, 6.4% reported that it would mean there would be no delay or loss of CD4 test results. Only 0.30% ($n = 2$) participants reported that they would not want this, because they needed time to consider the results.

Similarly, (b) in Table 1 presents participants' responses to the question about whether they would rather wait for their CD4 results or return another day. As with the first question ((a) in Table 1), the vast majority (96.4%) would rather wait for their CD4 test result, rather than return another day. There was some variation in reasons between the two clinics. Just over half (56.4%) of the sample reported wanting to get their results quickly and being able to start treatment; however, significantly less (48.1%) at Lancers than at Chesterville (64.7%) ($p < 0.0001$) reported this. Clinic accessibility was also a challenge, but this varied by clinic with significantly more patients at the Lancers Road (40.4%) than Chesterville PHC (24.7%) having difficulty with clinic accessibility ($p < 0.0001$). One in twenty (5.9%) at Lancers clinic reported they would not have the anxiety of waiting for their results if they received them within the day. An overall minority (3.4%) at both PHC clinics preferred CD4 test results on a different day.

Responses to whether participants knew what CD4 results meant are presented in (c) of Table 1. Over three-quarters (513/642 (79.9%)) had a good understanding of how a CD4 result would impact their health. Almost half (44.1%) emphasized how it assessed the level of CD4 cells in their blood, with some drawing on the language of "soldier cells" to describe CD4 cells. A quarter (23.5%) emphasized how the CD4 count was used to assess whether you were eligible to start treatment or the impact of treatment on health progression. A smaller group had a more general understanding around the CD4 count being a marker of HIV, with almost one in ten (9.8%) linking it to HIV viral load, and an assessment of health status. Just 2.5% emphasized that it assessed an HIV positive status. One-fifth (20.1%) reported that they had no understanding of what a CD4 test result meant.

Table 1. Patients' understanding and perceptions of the impact of a point-of-care (POC) laboratory provision of a CD4 test result at the primary healthcare (PHC) facility on their health.

		Reasons	Illustrative Example	Overall n = 642 (%)	Lancers Road PHC n = 322 * (%)	Chesterville PHC n = 320 * (%)	p	Z
(a) Are you happy to receive a CD4 test result on the same day? (n = 642)	Happy	Receive medical help	I like it because I will get assistance immediately if my results say so So that I know immediately if I'm supposed to start medication	474 (73.8)	237 (73.6)	237 (74.1)	0.9083	−0.12
		Saves time/money	I live far so it cost me a lot of money to come to the clinic So I won't have to take time off work to come to the clinic	125 (19.5)	67 (20.8)	58 (18.1)	0.3875	0.86
		No delay or loss of test results	It will avoid the loss of results and being drawn the blood again due to loss of them.	41 (6.4)	18 (5.6)	23 (7.2)	0.4075	−0.83
	Not Happy	Anxiety	I need time to get ready for the results	2 (0.3)	0	2 (0.6)	0.1645	−1.39
(b) Would you rather wait for a CD4 test result or return to clinic another day? * Not recorded for Lancers Road Clinic (n = 1)	Prefer to wait	Start Treatment	I would want to know if the treatment I am taking is working or not	362 (56.4)	155 (48.1)	207 (64.7)	<0.0001	−4.24
		Clinic inaccessibility	To save time and money for transport and I won't have to come back again for results since I hate being in the clinic I will save time, money and won't have to ask for leave at work for the second time	209 (32.6)	130 (40.4)	79 (24.7)	<0.0001	4.24
		No anxiety	If I wait for my result, I can deal with the stress same time I won't stress about the result if I get my result same day	33 (5.1)	19 (5.9)	14 (4.4)	0.3900	0.86
		No loss of samples	I like this because sometimes I come back for nothing, they tell me my blood was lost in the lab It can prevent loss of results	15 (2.3)	9 (2.8)	6 (1.9)	0.4518	0.75
	Not Wait	Not ready for results	It's better if I come back another day because I'm always rushing back to work Because there would be a long queue	22 (3.4)	8 (2.5)	14 (4.4)	0.1870	−1.32
(c) Do you know what a CD4 test result means?	Yes	CD4 cells/ Immune system	It tells how strong my CD4 cells I have Checking of soldier cells in the body It is your CD4 cell count.	283 (44.1)	153 (47.5)	130 (40.6)	0.0783	0.078
		Start treatment	It tells if you are ready to start treatment The results show the progress of the soldier cells in the body when taking medication.	151 (23.5)	69 (21.4)	82 (25.6)	0.2095	−1.26
		Viral load	It tells how much the virus is decreasing in the body	63 (9.8)	30 (9.3)	33 (10.3)	0.6700	−0.43
		HIV status	Tells me if I'm positive It tells me about HIV/AIDS	16 (2.5)	6 (1.9)	10 (3.1)	0.3300	−0.97
	No	Don't know		129 (20.1)	64 (19.9)	65 (20.3)	0.8994	0.899

Table 1. Cont.

(d) Are you ready to start ART if eligible? *Not recorded (n = 3 from each PHC)	Yes	Will live/make me better	It will help me from getting other infections Because I want to be healthy and live longer So I can be able to live longer So that I can protect myself and cannot spread the virus	286 (44.5)	147 (45.7)	139 (43.4)	0.5577	0.59
		Make me better in order to look after my family	Because I want to live longer as I have a family I'm ready because I don't want to die because I have children Because I have to, for the sake of my baby	7 (1.1)	6 (1.9)	1 (0.3)	0.0522	1.94
		Boost immune system/reduce viral load	I would start so that my CD4 levels stays high So it will increase my CD4 count	47 (7.3)	30 (9.3)	17 (5.3)	0.0515	1.95
		Ready		34 (5.3)	31 (9.6)	3 (0.9)	<0.0001	4.94
		No choice	Because I have no choice It's a must to start treatment whether I like it or not so that I can keep a healthy lifestyle	15 (2.3)	7 (2.2)	8 (2.5)	0.8019	−0.25
		Don't want to die	It's my life so I have to be responsible as if I don't take treatment, I will die I know if I don't start treatment if my CD4 is low, I will get sick and die so I will take it	17 (2.6)	11 (3.4)	6 (1.9)	0.2370	1.18
	No	Not ready	It will be hard because I haven't told anyone about my status because I know they won't accept it	23 (3.6)	10 (3.1)	13 (4.1)	0.4964	−0.68
		On ARVs. already		207 (32.2)	77 (23.9)	130 (40.6)	<0.0001	−4.53

Participants were asked if they had a CD4 test and were eligible for ART initiation, if they felt they were ready ((d) in Table 1). Over half (374/642) (58.2%) of patients were ready to start ART if they were eligible. Almost half (44.5%) of these responses were focused on living better and being healthier. Many of these suggested a good understanding of the potential benefits of being on ART. A very small group (1.1%) reported that it was so they could be healthier to look after their family, children, or baby, recognizing the social impact of ART, while 7.3% of responses focused on the biological benefit of ART and its impact on maintaining high levels of CD4. A small group (2.3%) reported that they would feel pressured to take ART if it was necessary. Lastly, some wanted to live and not die (2.6%). Only a small minority (3.6%) were not ready to take ARVs, giving reasons that the medication would make them feel sicker, they would forget to take them, they would require counselling prior to taking ARVs, and of stigma (anxious of what others would say).

There were 13 nurses interviewed, 5 at Lancers Road and 8 at Chesterville PHC, of whom 4/5 (80%) and 6/8 (80%) were females with a median age of 31 and 45.5 years, respectively. There were 3/5 (60%) and 1/8 (12.5%%) enrolled and 1/5 (20%) and 6/8 (75%) professional nurses at Lancers Road and Chesterville PHC, respectively, while 1/5 (20%) and 1/8 (12.5%) were staff nurses at each site.

Almost half of the nurses (46.2%) ((a) in Table 2) felt that it was beneficial for patients to get their CD4 result on the same day as it would facilitate knowing their disease progression, and this was felt to help with patients' management. Similarly, 7.7% of nurses felt it would enable patients to start ART quickly, again improving outcomes. Two nurses (15.4%) in the Chesterville PHC recognized the importance of being able to provide results on the same day for the convenience this provided to patients who may struggle to get in. One-third (30.8%) did not agree this was a good idea as the patient would have to take time off work (15.4%), and some patients were not ready for their results (15.4%). In particular, they raised the issue of being able to provide adequate counselling for patients as a potential challenge in providing results the same day.

Nurses also reflected on the impact on their workload of providing the CD4 results on the same day ((b) in Table 2). A third (30.8%) felt that it would reduce their workload as they could treat patients early and not have to see the same patients time and time again, and 15.4% of nurses also felt that it supported the patients and enabled them to start ART early by giving them clarity on their health.

In contrast, over half (53.8%) of nurses felt that it would increase the workload and not be beneficial; 30.8% described how this would increase their workload, as it would entail major administrative burdens, which would slow them down. Similarly, nearly a quarter (23.0%) were concerned that the other procedures to be completed before starting a person on ART would also lead to an increased workload.

Despite concerns about increased workload, the overwhelming majority of nurses emphasized that providing the CD4 results on the same day would help with clinical management of patients ((c) in Table 2). Almost half (46.2%) described how it would improve patient readiness, because patients would be provided with the information that they needed to understand their health. Closely associated with this would be how it may improve adherence (23.0%), with nurses being able to engage more closely with adherence counselling, as well as supporting patients in understanding the importance of adherence. One nurse (7.7%) emphasized how it would reduce follow-up visits by patients, therefore meaning that patients would not drop out. Those who were concerned about this were framed around the impact of immediate ART initiation, around requiring patients to have additional training and education (15.4%) in the context of shock of being newly diagnosed, and also requiring additional assistance from staff because of the additional tests that are needed before initiation.

Table 2. Nurses' understanding and perceptions of the impact of a POC laboratory provision of CD4 test results at the PHC facility with respect to patient workload, clinical management, and antiretroviral therapy (ART) administration/initiation.

Question	Response	Reasons	Illustrative Example	Overall n = 13 (%)	Lancers Road PHC n = 5 (%)	Chesterville PHC n = 8 (%)
(2a) Do you think it is beneficial for the patient to get their CD4 result on the same day?	Yes	Disease progression	They get to know how their immune system is doing. Because they will be informed about the progression of the disease in the body	6 (46.2)	4 (80)	2 (25)
		Convenience	Some patients work cannot afford to come to the clinic every second week. Other patients come when the clinic is very busy while they also work	2 (15.4)	0	2 (25)
		Start Treatment	Will speed up the process of initiating patients to ART and patients will get immediate care	1 (7.7)	0	1 (12.5)
	No	Time off work	If they have asked for time off at work for that day of blood draw, they might not get a chance to come another day to collect results	2 (15.4)	0	2 (25)
		Not ready for results	It's good and bad at the same time. It's good for someone who's been counselled well but others may not feel so good especially if they didn't even think of results	2 (15.4)	1 (20%)	1 (12.5)
(2b) What was the impact on your workload in giving CD4 results to the patient on the same day?	Beneficial	Reduce workload	It would make work easier and time saving because as a nurse, I won't see the patient over and over again about something that could be done in a day. It will be easy as you know that you will be dealing with patients and finish all procedures at once rather than calling them back.	4 (30.8)	1 (20)	3 (37.5)
		Treat patients early	It gives clarity on their CD4 count on whether they are starting ARVs, or not	2 (15.4)	1 (20)	1 (12.5)
	Not beneficial	Increase workload	It will increase my work load because there's too much administration when you initiate a person on treatment	4 (30.8)	3 (60)	1 (12.5)
		Complete all other procedures	It will increase workload; more staff like phlebotomists to take bloods. Patients will need to be prepared for ARV therapy, assess readiness and acceptance.	3 (23.0)	0	3 (37.5)

Table 2. Cont.

(2c) Does having a CD4 result on the same day help you with patient clinical management?	Yes	Patient readiness	Because the patients gets all the information and help he/she needs on the same day	6 (46.2)	2 (40)	4 (50)
		Adherence	It helps a lot to manage the patients who has low CD4 count	3 (23.0)	2 (40)	1 (12.5)
		Follow up visits	The patient won't have to come to the clinic for treatment so we won't lose the patients	1 (7.7)	0	1 (12.5)
		Assistance from other staff	It helps, but at the same time, it does not because there is a lot of tests that are done	1 (7.7)	0	1 (12.5)
	No	Training/Education	Yes, will definitely help, but on the other side, will be a disadvantage for patients who just tested positive; still a shock to them	2 (15.4)	1 (20)	1 (12.5)
(2d) Do you know what a CD4 test result mean?	Yes	Start treatment	Yes if patients have CD4 of 500 or less they are started on ART.	6 (46.2)	0	6 (75.0)
		Level of soldier cells	It tells me how high the level of soldier cells in the blood or how low the level of soldier cells in the blood	5 (38.5)	4 (80.0)	1 (12.5)
		Staging of HIV infection	It means patient is infected with the virus; gives me the picture of what stage the patient is in.	1 (7.7)	0	1 (12.5)
	No	Don't know		1 (7.7)	1 (20.0)	0
		Pregnant women	I managed the initiation of pregnant women as they are started on ARVs. immediately, regardless of their CD4 count	4 (30.8)	1 (20)	3 (37.5)
(2e) Were you able to administer ARVs. to the patient on the same day you had the CD4 test result?	Yes		Because I was directed by CD4 results, but with pregnant women, you provide ARVs. at the same time, regardless of CD4 count			
		Decrease Viral load	So it would help decrease the viral load	1 (7.7)	1 (20)	0
		Treatment initiation	The CD4 count result guided me into initiating a patient	1 (7.7)	1 (20)	0
	No	Require other blood tests	A patient is not initiated immediately; he/she needs to undergo some tests first. We need to check other diseases like TB, tests for liver and kidneys before initiating ARVS	4 (30.8)	2 (40)	2 (25)
		Patient education	That has not happened as yet in the clinic depending on the other things that need to be considered	1 (7.7)	0	1 (12.5)
		Not job description		1 (7.7)	0	1 (12.5)

*Not recorded in Chesterville PHC for (e) (n = 1)

The majority of nurses (92.3%) correctly interpreted a CD4 test result either as an indication of initiating treatment (46.2%), level of "soldier cells" (38.5%), or staging of HIV infection (7.7%), while 7.7% did not know the meaning of a CD4 test result ((d) in Table 2).

Nurses reported that they were able to administer ARVs. on the same day as giving a CD4 test ((e) in Table 2). Many (30.8%) reflected that this was because they had already done so for pregnant women. In addition, one (7.7%) reported that it would assist in reducing a patient's viral load. Finally, one nurse (7.7%) also noted that the CD4 count guided the initiation of treatment. A number of nurses raised concerns about initiation on the same day, and these were related to the need to have other blood tests done before ART could be prescribed (30.8%), while one nurse (7.7%) emphasized the importance of counselling. One nurse also highlighted that ART administration was not in their job description (7.7%).

4. Discussion

Overall, patients and nurses were positive about the CD4 POC testing and receiving CD4 results on the same day, with both practical benefits and medical benefits being described by both groups of people. Concerns expressed about receiving CD4 results on the same day were related to worry around the "shock" of tests results, and closely related to this, the need for counselling for new patients, and further tests, before ART initiation. Understanding this more broadly, POC testing was about providing important health information and enabling improved clinical management, as well as patients being able to understand their own health and start to take charge of it.

The majority of patients were happy to receive a same-day CD4 result and would rather wait for a short period of time for results. As they would receive medical intervention immediately, there would be no loss or delay of test results, saving them time, money, and clinic accessibility, and reducing anxiety. In the current study, among those who had received CD4 test results, the length of time was from 4 days to 4 weeks, through normal laboratory systems. Two-thirds of patients had a good understanding of the meaning of a CD4 test result and were ready to start ART if eligible.

Most nurses felt that a same-day CD4 test result was beneficial to the patient, would facilitate better clinical management, and would have an impact on either reducing or increasing their workload, including initiating ART, and most gave the correct explanation of the meaning of a CD4 test result.

Regardless of POC testing exposure or not, the high acceptability by patients and clinic staff of a same-day CD4 test result confirms findings from a feasibility and acceptability study of POC EID testing [9], finger-stick blood donation [10], and POC VL testing [24]. It suggests that currently there is limited fear attached to HIV disease due to the availability of life-saving medication, and it is considered a chronic condition with little stigma attached to it. The main motivation was receiving immediate treatment due to the elimination of loss or delay of results. This study corroborates findings of POC CD4 testing in South Africa and Zimbabwe where patients appreciated receiving rapid results for quicker clinical decision-making [30,31]. Numerous studies in African cohorts [12,32–35] have described poor rates of linkage to care for those eligible for ART due to several attrition challenges in the continuum of care pathway [22,36], including the unavailability of a CD4 test result [22,37].

A small minority preferred CD4 test results on a different day, most of whom were from the Chesterville PHC, reiterating that they were not ready to receive such information immediately. As has been described [11], they wanted to internalize and come to terms with what the results of the test meant in terms of implications for their health as well as not being able to wait due to a busy clinic and work commitment. The importance of this is that POC testing needs to be combined with supportive and effective counselling to ensure that it gives people space to adjust to the news they have just received, rather than it being provided on its own.

In this study, patients expressed several practical benefits of same-day POC CD4 testing: It would save time and days off work, cause less anxiety, and be a cost saver, which have been found to be important factors resulting in loss of linkage to care if not addressed [11]. Again, these are important findings about POC, no matter what the test is for, and they highlight structural constraints within the South African healthcare system and economy that POC testing may substantially overcome.

One of the barriers was clinic inaccessibility, particularly for patients attending the Lancers Road PHC. A significantly higher percentage of patients from the Chesterville PHC clinic received routine CD4 test results within 1–7 days due to the close proximity of the clinic facility, within walking distance in the community, compared to Lancers Road of 1–4 weeks where transport was required (data not shown).

Most (80%) patients correctly explained CD4 count results related to treatment initiation due to their immune status and facilitating decrease in viral load, while 20% of patients still did not understand the meaning of CD4 count results. Our study did not provide any education; however, in South Africa, there is a long history of CD4 count testing [38], particularly through the Treatment Action Campaign, which has encouraged treatment literacy focusing on CD4 testing. With the introduction of universal coverage in South Africa and VL monitoring [2], it has been recently suggested [24] that it would be important to increase awareness through education with respect to VL results. It is therefore important to ensure that information is not just provided on health outcomes for patients, but is also provided in understandable contexts with the meaning of it for their health.

The acceptability of ART initiation if eligible was high, with patients expressing the impact of life-saving ARVs. on making them feel better in order to take care of their family, longevity, and their action on their immune system and HIV virus, while a few gave no explanation. A minority felt they had no choice and were not ready.

Both professional and enrolled nurses felt that a same-day CD4 count result was beneficial to patients as it helped determine their disease progression in order to ascertain treatment initiation and patient convenience. However, one-third felt that some patients were not ready for same-day results to start treatment or would have to take time off work due to the turnaround of results.

With respect to workload, the opinions were divided. Half of the healthcare professionals felt that it would decrease their workload as patients would be treated early whereas the remainder felt this would increase their workload as all other tests would have to be completed before ART initiation, particularly at Lancers Road PHC, the reason being that it is an extremely busy clinic with a heavy patient load [8].

With respect to clinical management, professional nurses felt that a same-day CD4 test result would facilitate patient readiness, adherence to ART, and fewer follow-up visits. We concur with findings from two qualitative studies, one from South Africa [39] and the other from Uganda [40], where healthcare workers found that POC testing resulted in earlier interventions and reduced burden of patient clinic visits. Only a minority in this study felt that they needed extra assistance and further training and education. All but one nurse (staff nurse) did not correctly interpret the meaning of a CD4 result, as this was not in her job description. Half of the nurses felt it was beneficial to have a POC CD4 count as it would facilitate ART initiation in pregnant women, as was found in a study from Zimbabwe [30]. Our findings are similar to Spooner et al. (2019) [9], in that the remainder were concerned that other tests were still required before ART initiation.

Although current programmes could be enhanced by the introduction of POC testing [41,42] to address some existing challenges [43], it has been suggested [44,45] that certain factors need to be considered before POC implementation: Clinic flows, diagnostic accuracy, staff training, quality control, and turnaround times. In South Africa, multiple strategies [46] have previously been used to overcome high patient burden and staff shortages [7] with respect to rapid HIV testing. The United Nations International Children's Emergency Fund (UNICEF) have described the steps necessary for the incorporation of POC diagnostic testing into national health laboratory systems [47].

The strength of this study is the large patient sample size, collection of both quantitative and qualitative data from the general PHC population, its being undertaken in two different geographic settings, and the POC testing experience.

The limitations are the small sample size of healthcare professionals and the lack of inclusion of other stakeholders for their insights into the advantages and disadvantages of POC testing from their perspective. The qualitative data were from a closed-caption set of questions, and few respondents wrote more than a short sentence as an answer to any question. While in-depth qualitative interviews and focus-group discussions can generate more detailed information and understanding of a topic under consideration, the qualitative survey did allow for a large number of views to be generated from patients and some form of quantification to be done to describe the overall perceptions of patients.

5. Conclusions

The high patient and nurse acceptability of POC CD4 testing and their grasp of the immediate health and structural benefits (time, cost savings, and time off work) in the former and clinical management in the latter lends itself to undertaking implementation studies in the future in order to address barriers [24]. This is particularly important for POC VL testing, which is used as the hallmark for treatment success [48,49], so that the third 90 of The Joint United Nations Programme on HIV and AIDS (UNAIDS) 2020 target [50] can be achieved. It also has implications for POC testing more widely, suggesting that patients and healthcare providers recognize its wide-ranging benefit.

Author Contributions: S.R. provided management of the research project; A.G. provided management and analysis of the qualitative data and write-up; N.N. and N.J. provided access to the PHC clinics; T.R. provided statistical support; G.R. provided funding; E.S., A.C., and P.K. conceptualized the proposal; S.R., A.G., and P.K. contributed to writing the final draft. All authors have read and agreed to the published version of the manuscript.

Funding: This study was supported by the Metropolitan and Momentum Investment (MMI) Foundation (corporate social investment arm of MMI Holdings) to G.R. A.G. was funded by the South African Medical Research Council.

Acknowledgments: The authors thank Phumla Ndamase, Thabsile Maluleka, Siziphiwe Dayi, Wendy Mfati, Silindile Khubeka, and Silindile Shangase for undertaking the informed consent and administration of questionnaires. We also thank the clinical and administrative staff at the Lancers Road and Chesterville PHC clinics whose cooperation is gratefully acknowledged.

Conflicts of Interest: The authors declare that they have no financial or personal relationship(s) that may have inappropriately influenced them in writing this article.

References

1. Statistics South Africa (STATSA). Statistical Release P0302: Mid-Year Population Estimates. 2019. Available online: http://www.statssa.gov.za/?p=12362 (accessed on 31 August 2019).
2. National Department of Health South Africa. Re: Implementation of the Universal Test and Treat Strategy for HIV Positive Patients and Differentiated Care for Stable Patients. 2016. Available online: https://sahivsoc.org/Files/22%208%2016%20Circular%20UTT%20%20%20Decongestion%20CCMT%20Directorate.pdf (accessed on 14 October 2019).
3. World Health Organization. *Guideline on When to Start Antiretroviral Therapy and on Pre-Exposure Prophylaxis for HIV*; WHO: Geneva, Switzerland, 2015; Available online: https://apps.who.int/iris/bitstream/handle/10665/186275/9789241509565_eng.pdf (accessed on 30 September 2019).
4. UNAIDS. South Africa UNAIDS 2017. Available online: https://www.unaids.org/en/regionscountries/countries/southafrica (accessed on 5 August 2018).
5. Maillacheruvu, P.; McDuff, E. South Africa's Return to Primary Care: The Struggles and Strides of the Primary Health Care System. *J. Glob. Health* **2014**. Available online: https://www.ghjournal.org/south-africas-return-to-primary-care-the-struggles-and-strides-of-the-primary-health-care-system/ (accessed on 1 October 2019).
6. Gous, N.M.; Berrie, L.; Dabula, P.; Stevens, W. South Africa's experience with provision of quality HIV diagnostic services. *Afr. J. Lab. Med.* **2016**, *5*, 436. [CrossRef] [PubMed]
7. Engel, N.; Davids, M.; Blankvoort, N.; Pai, N.P.; Dheda, K.; Pai, M. Compounding diagnostic delays: A qualitative study of point-of-care testing in South Africa. *Trop. Med. Int. Health* **2015**, *20*, 493–500. [CrossRef] [PubMed]

8. Cloete, M.C.; Hampton, J.; Chetty, T.; Ngomane, T.; Spooner, E.; Zako, L.M.G.; Reddy, S.; Reddy, T.; Luthuli, N.; Ngobese, H.; et al. Evaluation of a health system intervention to improve virological management in an antiretroviral programme at a municipal clinic in central Durban. *South. Afr. J. HIV Med.* **2019**, *20*, 985. [CrossRef] [PubMed]
9. Spooner, E.; Govender, K.; Reddy, T.; Ramjee, G.; Mbadi, N.; Singh, S.; Coutsoudis, A. Point-of-care HIV testing best practice for early infant diagnosis: An implementation study. *BMC Public Health* **2019**, *19*, 731. [CrossRef] [PubMed]
10. Daneau, G.; Gous, N.; Scott, L.; Potgieter, J.; Kestens, L.; Stevens, W. Human Immunodeficiency Virus (HIV)-Infected Patients Accept Finger Stick Blood Collection for Point-Of-Care CD4 Testing. *PLoS ONE* **2016**, *11*, e0161891. [CrossRef] [PubMed]
11. Govindasamy, D.; Ford, N.; Kranzer, K. Risk factors, barriers and facilitators for linkage to antiretroviral therapy care: A systematic review. *AIDS* **2012**, *26*, 2059–2067. [CrossRef]
12. Jani, I.V.; Sitoe, N.E.; Alfai, E.R.; Chongo, P.L.; Quevedo, J.I.; Rocha, B.M.; Lehe, J.D.; Peter, T.F. Effect of point-of-care CD4 cell count tests on retention of patients and rates of antiretroviral therapy initiation in primary health clinics: An observational cohort study. *Lancet* **2011**, *378*, 1572–1579. [CrossRef]
13. Vojnov, L.; Markby, J.; Boeke, C.; Harris, L.; Ford, N.; Peter, T. POC CD4 Testing Improves Linkage to HIV Care and Timeliness of ART Initiation in a Public Health Approach: A Systematic Review and Meta-Analysis. *PLoS ONE* **2016**, *11*, e0155256. [CrossRef]
14. Stevens, W.S.; Gous, N.M.; MacLeod, W.B.; Long, L.C.; Variava, E.; Martinson, N.A.; Sanne, I.; Osih, R.; Scott, L.E. Multidisciplinary Point-of-Care Testing in South African Primary Health Care Clinics Accelerates HIV ART Initiation but Does Not Alter Retention in Care. *J. Acquir. Immune Defic. Syndr.* **2017**, *76*, 65–73. [CrossRef]
15. Naidoo, P.; du Toit, E.; Dunbar, R.; Lombard, C.; Caldwell, J.; Detjen, A.; Squire, S.B.; Enarson, D.A.; Beyers, N. A comparison of multidrug-resistant tuberculosis treatment commencement times in MDRTBPlus line probe assay and Xpert(R) MTB/RIF-based algorithms in a routine operational setting in Cape Town. *PLoS ONE* **2014**, *9*, e103328. [CrossRef]
16. Hyle, E.P.; Jani, I.V.; Lehe, J.; Su, A.E.; Wood, R.; Quevedo, J.; Losina, E.; Bassett, I.V.; Pei, P.P.; Paltiel, A.D.; et al. The clinical and economic impact of point-of-care CD4 testing in Mozambique and other resource-limited settings: A cost-effectiveness analysis. *PLoS Med.* **2014**, *11*, e1001725. [CrossRef] [PubMed]
17. Ciaranello, A.L.; Myer, L.; Kelly, K.; Christensen, S.; Daskilewicz, K.; Doherty, K.; Bekker, L.G.; Hou, T.; Wood, R.; Francke, J.A.; et al. Point-of-care CD4 testing to inform selection of antiretroviral medications in South African antenatal clinics: A cost-effectiveness analysis. *PLoS ONE* **2015**, *10*, e0117751. [CrossRef] [PubMed]
18. Pai, N.P.; Vadnais, C.; Denkinger, C.; Engel, N.; Pai, M. Point-of-care testing for infectious diseases: Diversity, complexity, and barriers in low- and middle-income countries. *PLoS Med.* **2012**, *9*, e1001306. [CrossRef] [PubMed]
19. Jani, I.V.; Peter, T.F. How point-of-care testing could drive innovation in global health. *N. Engl. J. Med.* **2013**, *368*, 2319–2324. [CrossRef]
20. Stime, K.J.; Garrett, N.; Sookrajh, Y.; Dorward, J.; Dlamini, N.; Olowolagba, A.; Sharma, M.; Barnabas, R.V.; Drain, P.K. Clinic flow for STI, HIV, and TB patients in an urban infectious disease clinic offering point-of-care testing services in Durban, South Africa. *BMC Health Serv. Res.* **2018**, *18*, 363. [CrossRef]
21. Munkhuu, B.; Liabsuetrakul, T.; McNeil, E.; Janchiv, R. Feasibility of one-stop antenatal syphilis screening in Ulaanbaatar, Mongolia: Women and providers perspectives. *Southeast Asian J. Trop. Med. Public Health* **2009**, *40*, 861–870.
22. Wynberg, E.; Cooke, G.; Shroufi, A.; Reid, S.D.; Ford, N. Impact of point-of-care CD4 testing on linkage to HIV care: A systematic review. *J. Int. AIDS Soc.* **2014**, *17*, 18809. [CrossRef]
23. Jani, I.V.; Meggi, B.; Loquiha, O.; Tobaiwa, O.; Mudenyanga, C.; Zitha, A.; Mutsaka, D.; Mabunda, N.; Vubil, A.; Bollinger, T.; et al. Effect of point-of-care early infant diagnosis on antiretroviral therapy initiation and retention of patients. *AIDS* **2018**, *32*, 1453–1463. [CrossRef]
24. Msimango, L.; Gibbs, A.; Shozi, H.; Ngobese, H.; Humphries, H.; Drain, P.K.; Garrett, N.; Dorward, J. *Acceptability of Point-Of-Care Viral Load Testing to Facilitate Differentiated Care: A Qualitative Assessment of People Living with HIV and Healthcare Workers in South Africa*; International AIDS Society: Mexico City, Mexico, 2019.

25. Skhosana, M.; Reddy, S.; Reddy, T.; Ntoyanto, S.; Spooner, E.; Ramjee, G.; Ngomane, N.; Coutsoudis, A.; Kiepiela, P. PIMA point-of-care testing for CD4 counts in predicting antiretroviral initiation in HIV-infected individuals in KwaZulu-Natal, Durban, South Africa. *South Afr. J. HIV Med.* **2016**, *17*, 444.
26. Reddy, S.; Ntoyanto, S.; Sakadavan, Y.; Reddy, T.; Mahomed, S.; Dlamini, M.; Spooner, B.; Ramjee, G.; Coutsoudis, A.; Ngomane, N.; et al. Detecting Mycobacterium tuberculosis using the loop-mediated isothermal amplification test in South Africa. *Int. J. Tuberc. Lung Dis.* **2017**, *21*, 1154–1160. [CrossRef] [PubMed]
27. The Logic of Qualitative Survey Research and its Position in the Field of Social Research Methods. Available online: http://www.qualitative-research.net/index.php/fqs/article/view/1450/2946. (accessed on 1 November 2019).
28. Sub Place Chesterville. Census. 2011. Available online: https://census2011.adrianfrith.com/place/599054041 (accessed on 30 September 2019).
29. South African Department of Health. The South African Antiretroviral Treatment Guidelines. 2010. Available online: https://apps.who.int/medicinedocs/documents/s19153en/s19153en.pdf (accessed on 30 September 2019).
30. Mtapuri-Zinyowera, S.; Chiyaka, E.T.; Mushayi, W.; Musuka, G.; Naluyinda-Kitabire, F.; Mushavi, A.; Chikwasha, V. PIMA Point of Care CD4+ Cell Count Machines in Remote MNCH Settings: Lessons Learned from Seven Districts in Zimbabwe. *Infect. Dis.* **2013**, *6*, 51–60. [CrossRef] [PubMed]
31. Jain, K.; Mshweshwe-Pakela, N.T.; Charalambous, S.; Mabuto, T.; Hoffmann, C.J. Enhancing value and lowering costs of care: A qualitative exploration of a randomized linkage to care intervention in South Africa. *AIDS Care* **2019**, *31*, 481–488. [CrossRef]
32. Fox, M.P.; Rosen, S. Patient retention in antiretroviral therapy programs up to three years on treatment in sub-Saharan Africa, 2007–2009: Systematic review. *Trop. Med. Int. Health* **2010**, *15* (Suppl. 1), 1–15. [CrossRef] [PubMed]
33. Larson, B.A.; Schnippel, K.; Ndibongo, B.; Xulu, T.; Brennan, A.T.; Long, L.C.; Fox, M.P.; Rosen, S. Rapid point-of-care CD4 testing at mobile HIV testing sites to increase linkage to care: An evaluation of a pilot program in South Africa. *J. Acquir. Immune Defic. Syndr.* **2012**, *61*, e13–e17. [CrossRef] [PubMed]
34. Rosen, S.; Fox, M.P. Retention in HIV care between testing and treatment in sub-Saharan Africa: A systematic review. *PLoS Med.* **2011**, *8*, e1001056. [CrossRef] [PubMed]
35. Mugglin, C.; Estill, J.; Wandeler, G.; Bender, N.; Egger, M.; Gsponer, T.; Keiser, O.; IeDEA Southern Africa. Loss to programme between HIV diagnosis and initiation of antiretroviral therapy in sub-Saharan Africa: Systematic review and meta-analysis. *Trop. Med. Int. Health* **2012**, *17*, 1509–1520. [CrossRef]
36. Patten, G.E.; Wilkinson, L.; Conradie, K.; Isaakidis, P.; Harries, A.D.; Edginton, M.E.; De Azevedo, V.; van Cutsem, G. Impact on ART initiation of point-of-care CD4 testing at HIV diagnosis among HIV-positive youth in Khayelitsha, South Africa. *J. Int. AIDS Soc.* **2013**, *16*, 18518. [CrossRef]
37. Losina, E.; Bassett, I.V.; Giddy, J.; Chetty, S.; Regan, S.; Walensky, R.P.; Ross, D.; Scott, C.A.; Uhler, L.M.; Katz, J.N.; et al. The "ART" of linkage: Pre-treatment loss to care after HIV diagnosis at two PEPFAR sites in Durban, South Africa. *PLoS ONE* **2010**, *5*, e9538. [CrossRef]
38. Paparini, S.; Rhodes, T. The biopolitics of engagement and the HIV cascade of care: A synthesis of the literature on patient citizenship and antiretroviral therapy. *Crit. Public Health* **2016**, *26*, 501–517. [CrossRef]
39. Mashamba-Thompson, T.P.; Jama, N.A.; Sartorius, B.; Drain, P.K.; Thompson, R.M. Implementation of Point-of-Care Diagnostics in Rural Primary Healthcare Clinics in South Africa: Perspectives of Key Stakeholders. *Diagnostics* **2017**, *7*, 3. [CrossRef] [PubMed]
40. Rasti, R.; Nanjebe, D.; Karlstrom, J.; Muchunguzi, C.; Mwanga-Amumpaire, J.; Gantelius, J.; Mårtensson, A.; Rivas, L.; Galban, F.; Reuterswärd, P.; et al. Health care workers' perceptions of point-of-care testing in a low-income country-A qualitative study in Southwestern Uganda. *PLoS ONE* **2017**, *12*, e0182005. [CrossRef]
41. Mashamba-Thompson, T.P.; Sartorius, B.; Drain, P.K. Point-of-Care Diagnostics for Improving Maternal Health in South Africa. *Diagnostics* **2016**, *6*, 31. [CrossRef] [PubMed]
42. Mashamba-Thompson, T.P.; Sartorius, B.; Drain, P.K. Operational assessment of point-of-care diagnostics in rural primary healthcare clinics of KwaZulu-Natal, South Africa: A cross-sectional survey. *BMC Health Serv. Res.* **2018**, *18*, 380. [CrossRef] [PubMed]

43. Gous, N.; Takle, J.; Oppenheimer, A.; Schooley, A. Racing for results: Lessons learnt in improving the efficiency of HIV viral load and early infant diagnosis result delivery from laboratory to clinic. *Expert Rev. Mol. Diagn.* **2018**, *18*, 789–795. [CrossRef]
44. Pai, N.P.; Wilkinson, S.; Deli-Houssein, R.; Vijh, R.; Vadnais, C.; Behlim, T.; Steben, M.; Engel, N.; Wong, T. Barriers to Implementation of Rapid and Point-of-Care Tests for Human Immunodeficiency Virus Infection: Findings from a Systematic Review (1996–2014). *Point Care* **2015**, *14*, 81–87. [CrossRef]
45. Jones, C.H.; Howick, J.; Roberts, N.W.; Price, C.P.; Heneghan, C.; Plüddemann, A.; Thompson, M. Primary care clinicians' attitudes towards point-of-care blood testing: A systematic review of qualitative studies. *BMC Fam. Pract.* **2013**, *14*, 117. [CrossRef]
46. Engel, N.; Davids, M.; Blankvoort, N.; Dheda, K.; Pant, P.N.; Pai, M. Making HIV testing work at the point of care in South Africa: A qualitative study of diagnostic practices. *BMC Health Serv. Res.* **2017**, *17*, 408. [CrossRef]
47. UNICEF: Key Considerations for Introducing New HIV Point-of-Care Diagnostic Technologies in National Health Systems. 2017. Available online: http://www.childrenandaidsorg/poc-toolkit-page. (accessed on 17 September 2019).
48. Gupta, R.K.; Jordan, M.R.; Sultan, B.J.; Hill, A.; Davis, D.H.; Gregson, J.; Sawyer, A.W.; Hamers, R.L.; Ndembi, N.; Pillay, D.; et al. Global trends in antiretroviral resistance in treatment-naive individuals with HIV after rollout of antiretroviral treatment in resource-limited settings: A global collaborative study and meta-regression analysis. *Lancet* **2012**, *380*, 1250–1258. [CrossRef]
49. Estill, J.; Aubrière, C.; Egger, M.; Johnson, L.; Wood, R.; Garone, D.; Gsponer, T.; Wandeler, G.; Boulle, A.; Davies, M.A.; et al. Viral load monitoring of antiretroviral therapy, cohort viral load and HIV transmission in Southern Africa: A mathematical modelling analysis. *AIDS* **2012**, *26*, 1403–1413. [CrossRef]
50. UNAIDS. Fast-Track Ending the AIDS Epidemic by 2030. 2014. Available online: http://unaids.org/en/resources/documents/2014/JC2686 (accessed on 5 August 2019).

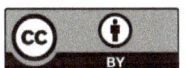

© 2020 by the authors. Licensee MDPI, Basel, Switzerland. This article is an open access article distributed under the terms and conditions of the Creative Commons Attribution (CC BY) license (http://creativecommons.org/licenses/by/4.0/).

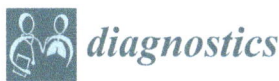

Article

Impact of Implementing Antenatal Syphilis Point-of-Care Testing on Maternal Mortality in KwaZulu-Natal, South Africa: An Interrupted Time Series Analysis

Tivani P. Mashamba-Thompson [1], Paul K. Drain [2,3,4,5], Desmond Kuupiel [1,*] and Benn Sartorius [1,6]

[1] Discipline of Public Health Medicine, School of Nursing and Public Health, University of KwaZulu-Natal, Durban 4041, South Africa; Mashamba-Thompson@ukzn.ac.za (T.P.M.-T.); benn.sartorius1@lshtm.ac.uk (B.S.)
[2] International Clinical Research Center, Department of Global Health, University of Washington, Seattle, WA 98195-7965, USA; pkdrain@uw.edu
[3] Division of Infectious Diseases, Department of Medicine, University of Washington, Seattle, WA 98195-7965, USA
[4] Department of Epidemiology, University of Washington, Seattle, WA 98195-7965, USA
[5] Department of Surgery, Harvard University, Massachusetts General Hospital, Boston, MA 02114, USA
[6] Faculty of Infectious and Tropical Diseases, London School of Hygiene and Tropical Medicine, London WC1H 9SH, UK
* Correspondence: desmondkuupiel98@hotmail.com

Received: 29 September 2019; Accepted: 5 December 2019; Published: 10 December 2019

Abstract: Background: Syphilis infection has been associated with an increased risk of HIV infection during pregnancy which poses greater risk for maternal mortality, and antenatal syphilis point-of-care (POC) testing has been introduced to improve maternal and child health outcomes. There is limited evidence on the impact of syphilis POC testing on maternal outcomes in high HIV prevalent settings. We used syphilis POC testing as a model to evaluate the impact of POC diagnostics on the improvement of maternal mortality in KwaZulu-Natal, South Africa. Methods: We extracted 132 monthly data points on the number of maternal deaths in facilities and number of live births in facilities for 12 tertiary healthcare facilities in KwaZulu-Natal (KZN), South Africa from 2004 to 2014 from District Health Information System (DHIS) health facility archived. We employed segmented Poisson regression analysis of interrupted time series to assess the impact of the exposure on maternal mortality ratio (MMR) before and after the implementation of antenatal syphilis POC testing. We processed and analyzed data using Stata Statistical Software: Release 13. (Stata, Corp LP, College Station, TX, USA). Results: The provincial average annual maternal mortality ratio (MMR) was estimated at 176.09 ± 43.92 ranging from a minimum of 68.48 to maximum of 225.49 per 100,000 live births. The data comprised 36 temporal points before the introduction of syphilis POC test exposure and 84 after the introduction in primary health care clinics in KZN. The average annual MMR for KZN from 2004 to 2014 was estimated at 176.09 ± 43.92. A decrease in MMR level was observed during 2008 after syphilis POC test implementation, followed by a rise during 2009. Analysis of the MMR trend estimates a significant 1.5% increase in MMR trends during the period before implementation and 1.3% increase after implementation of syphilis POC testing ($p < 0.001$). Conclusion: Although our finding suggests a brief reduction in the MMR trend after the implementation of antenatal syphilis POC testing, a continued increase in syphilis rates is seen in KwaZulu-Natal, South Africa. The study used one of the most powerful quasi-experimental research methods, segmented Poisson regression analysis of interrupted time series to model the impact of syphilis POC on maternal outcome. The study finding requires confirmation by use of more rigorous primary study design.

Keywords: syphilis; point-of-care testing; maternal mortality; interrupted time series; segmented regression analysis

1. Background

South Africa accounts for 18% of global HIV infections, with approximately 6.7 million people infected [1]. There are almost 1000 new HIV infections per day, the majority of which are heterosexually transmitted [2]. The 2019 Statistics South Africa National Estimates report shows an ongoing increase in total number of persons living with HIV in South Africa [3]. This number has increased from an estimated 4.64 million in 2002 to 7.97 million by 2019 [3]. The report also shows that over a fifth of South African women in their reproductive ages (15–49 years) are HIV positive [3]. A recent report on maternal health indicates that non-pregnancy-related infections due to HIV/AIDS contribute to 43.7% of the total maternal mortality in South Africa [4]. The 2014 Amnesty International report on maternal health in KwaZulu-Natal (KZN) and Mpumalanga 2008–2010 highlights the barriers, such as poor access to health care, resulting in women and girls delaying or avoiding antenatal care in and maternal deaths [5].

Point-of-care (POC) testing is one innovation that has been proven to help improve healthcare access by enabling early diagnosis and linkage to care [6]. Syphilis point-of-care (POC) testing is provided as part of the routine antenatal services in South Africa. This was implemented to help improve healthcare access and neonatal health outcomes [7–11]. The introduction of syphilis POC testing has been shown to be effective in strengthening health systems by improving access to quality-assured prenatal screening and saving new-born lives in resource-limited settings [12,13]. The results of our survey which was aimed at determining the availability and utility of POC diagnostics in rural KZN has demonstrated that syphilis testing was available and used in all districts, but the level of availability and use varied from clinic to clinic [14]. Overall 50% (CI: 60–40%) of the clinics used syphilis tests [14].

Syphilis infection has been associated with HIV through facilitating HIV transmission and the combination of syphilis, particularly during pregnancy [9,15]. Early detection of *Treponema pallidum* and prompt penicillin treatment for pregnant women who test positive have been shown to be effective in reducing adverse pregnancy outcomes [16–18]. Syphilis has also been demonstrated to increase HIV viral load and decrease CD4 cell counts in HIV-infected patients with syphilis infections [19,20]. Atypical presentations of early syphilis, rapid progression to tertiary syphilis, treatment failures, and more frequent cases of neurosyphilis have been reported amongst HIV-infected populations [15]. This is a concern for low- and middle-income countries, such as South Africa, that have high rates of HIV-related maternal mortality [5,21].

Despite this, little is known about the impact of syphilis POC testing on maternal mortality, particularly in high HIV settings. The results of our systematic review revealed that there is limited evidence on the impact of syphilis POC diagnostics on maternal outcomes of HIV-infected women [4]. The main aim of this study is to determine the impact of antenatal syphilis POC diagnostics on maternal mortality in KwaZulu-Natal, South Africa, using a time series study design. Demonstrating the impact of currently used syphilis POC testing on maternal mortality will enable us to determine whether or not the introduction of syphilis POC diagnostics has had any tangible effect on key maternal outcomes to enable justification of the need for syphilis POC diagnostic scale-up in settings that lack laboratory infrastructure such as rural antenatal health clinics.

2. Methodology

This study was conducted as part of a large implementation research study aimed at evaluating the accessibility and utility of POC diagnostics for maternal health in rural South Africa primary healthcare clinics (PHC) in order to generate a model framework of implementation of POC diagnostics in rural South African clinics [22].

2.1. Study Design, Population, and Location

We conducted a retrospective study using monthly MMR data from all 11 districts in KZN province, South Africa from 2004 to 2014. KZN province was purposively selected due to the high prevalence of HIV and high maternal mortality. A quasi-experimental approach is a powerful approach for evaluating effects of presence and absence of an exposure on outcomes [23,24].

2.2. Exposure

As reported by the KZN Department of Health, Rapid Plasma Reagin (RPR; Biotec Lab, Suffolk, UK) syphilis POC testing was implemented as part of the routine diagnostic tests for antenatal care in primary healthcare facilities during 2007. Syphilis POC test forms one the routine antenatal diagnostic tests offered by nurses at PHC clinics. Prior to the introduction of syphilis POC testing in this region, syphilis testing was performed at the laboratory associated with the health facility using Lovibond (Orbeco-Hellige, FL, USA) and Rapid Plasma Reagin (RPR; Biotec Lab, Suffolk, UK), respectively.

2.3. Data Extraction

We extracted archived records on the number of annual live births and number of maternal deaths in KZN from existing routine data from the District Health Information System (DHIS; Table S1). Earlier studies of the DHIS system have reported that the quality of the data, including those used to track prevention of mother to child transmission (PMTCT) care, is suboptimal [25]. Following these reports, in 2008 the KwaZulu-Natal Department of Health, the University of KwaZulu-Natal, and the Institute for Health care Improvement launched a large-scale effort, entitled the 20,000+ Partnership, to improve the completeness and accuracy of the public health data routinely recorded in the DHIS implemented between May 2008 and March 2009 [26]. This exposure has led to improved data reliability and validity [26].

We extracted data from KZN tertiary facilities that contained data on number of maternal deaths in the facility and number of live births in the facility from 2004 to 2014. Data prior to 2004, after 2014, and other data that were not relevant to maternal health were excluded. The DHIS presents district level data on all the maternal health indicators required to calculated MMR. We extracted district level data on number of maternal deaths in facilities and number of live births in facilities to help us calculate MMR.

2.4. Data analysis

We processed and analyzed data using Stata Statistical Software: Release 13. (College Station, TX: StataCorp LP). The exposure (syphilis POC test) was implemented as part of the routine diagnostic tests for antenatal care in primary healthcare facilities during 2007. Hence, we conducted a pre-post analysis of this exposure. Estimation of the impact of syphilis POC diagnostics on overall MMR in all KZN districts was conducted using the exposure time series approach [27]. We used the Poisson formulation approach, given maternal death count (with live births as the exposure) to estimate changes in levels and trends in maternal deaths during the period before and after implementation of syphilis POC testing in KZN, using the following equation:

$$\hat{Y}_t = \log(L_t) + \beta_0 + \beta_1 \times \text{time} + \beta_2 \times \text{exposure} + \beta_3 \times \text{time after exposure} + e_t$$

Where $\hat{Y}_t$ is the outcome (maternal deaths); L_t is the live birth count; time indicates the number of months from the start of the series; exposure is the dummy variable taking the values 0 in the pre-exposure segment and 1 in the post-exposure segment; time after exposure is 0 in the pre-exposure segment and counts the months in the post-exposure segment at time t; the coefficient β_0 estimates the base level of the outcome (MMR) at the beginning of the series; β_1 estimates the base trend, i.e., the change in outcome per month in the pre-exposure segment; β_2 estimates the change in level of MMR on the post-exposure segment; β_3 estimates the change in trend in MMR in the post-exposure segment; and e_t estimates the error

We used line graphs to visually display the series over time namely, one curve represented the observed MMR by year and month while a second line displayed the predicted line from the segmented regression model. Model coefficients were exponentiated to represent relative risks (RR).

2.5. Ethics Statement

We received full ethical approval and permission to conduct this study from the KZN Department of Heath (DoH) Ethics Committee (HRKM 40/15). We also received ethical approval for the current study from the University of KwaZulu-Natal (UKZN) Biomedical Research Ethics Committee (BE484/14). Data used in this study was extracted from the national database. Therefore, patient informed consent was not required.

3. Results

Summary of the Study Population and Sample Size

A total of 132 consecutive monthly MMR data points from 12 tertiary healthcare facilities from all 11 KZN districts were assessed from 2004 to 2014. The data comprised of 36 temporal points before the introduction of syphilis POC test exposure and 84 after the introduction in primary health care clinics (Table S1). The average annual MMR for KZN from 2004 to 2014 was estimated at 176.09 ± 43.92 ranging from a minimum of 68.48 to a maximum of 225.49 (Table 1). Table 1 shows a drop in MMR by 34.2% in 2008 followed by a 35.5% rise in 2009.

Table 1. Maternal mortality rate by year for all KwaZulu-Natal.

Year	Number of Maternal Deaths in Facility	Number of Live Births in Facility	Maternal Mortality Ratio Per 100,000 Live Births
2004	208	159712	130.23
2005	259	145617	177.86
2006	371	171230	216.67
2007	337	168580	199.91
2008	120	175227	68.48
2009	324	167847	193.03
2010	291	167544	173.69
2011	378	167637	225.49
2012	312	164322	189.87
2013	256	163411	156.66
2014	254	159484	159.26

Figure 1 shows an annual increase in maternal mortality ratio (MMR) level from 2004 to 2014, with a prominent drop in MMR level in 2008. Figure 2 shows the average and monthly fluctuations in MMR levels. A 35% decrease in MMR level was estimated during implementation of the syphilis POC test ($p < 0.001$; Table 2).

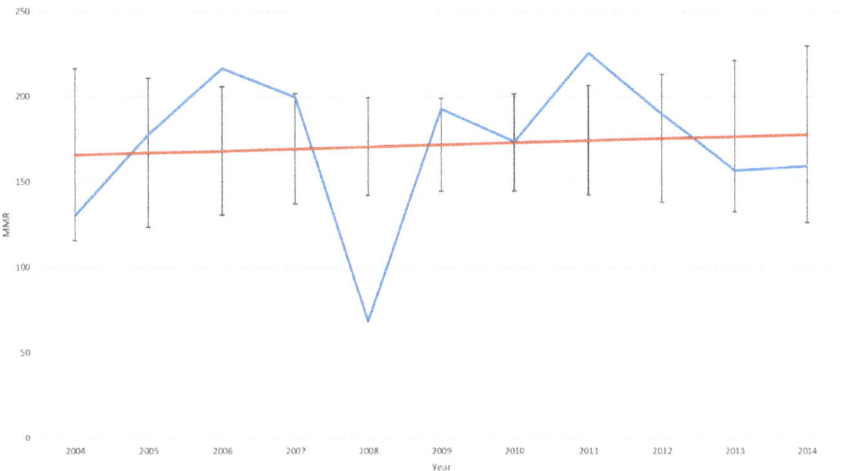

Figure 1. Maternal mortality ratio (MMR) by year for all KwaZulu-Natal with trend line (and 95% CI) excluding 2005 outlier (detected from raw data).

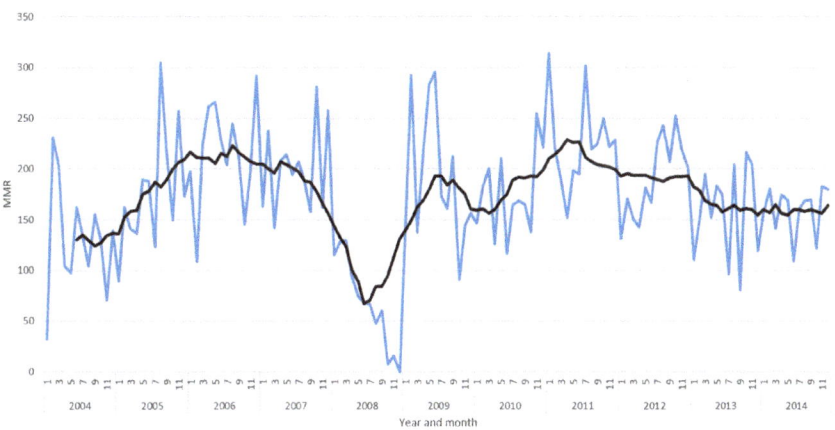

Figure 2. Maternal mortality ratio (MMR) by year for all KZN by month with 12 months moving average line (black).

Table 2. Longitudinal analysis of monthly maternal mortality using a fully segmented Poisson regression model.

Full Segmented Regression Model	RR	95% CI		p Value
		Lower	Upper	
A_0—Intercept i (2007, introduction of POC testing)	0.001	0.001	0.001	—
A_1—Baseline trend (before introduction of syphilis POC testing)	1.015	1.01	1.021	<0.001
A_2—Level change after introduction of syphilis POC testing	0.653	0.567	0.752	<0.001
A_3—Trend change introduction of syphilis POC testing	0.987	0.981	0.992	<0.001

Table 2 and Figure 3 depict results from the segmented Poisson regression (interrupted time series) model. Based on the smoothed line plots and the reported relative risk (RR), there is a significant decrease in the monthly MMR before and after the syphilis POC testing exposure in KZN (35%). A significant 1.5% increase in MMR was observed ($p < 0.001$) before the introduction of syphilis POC testing exposure (2004–2006). MMR during the period after the introduction of syphilis POC testing exposure (2008–2014) rose significantly by 1.3% every month ($p < 0.001$).

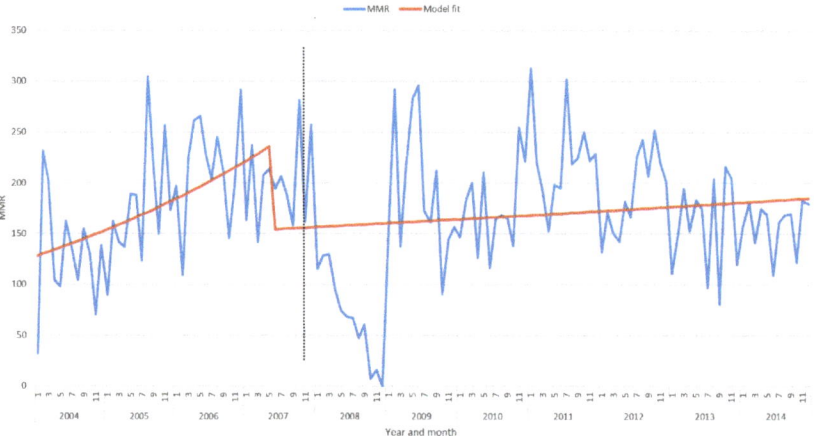

Figure 3. MMR by year for all KZN by month with fitted interrupted time series segmented regression line (exposure implementation represented by vertical dotted line).

4. Discussion

Our study shows that implementation of antenatal syphilis POC tests has the potential to improve maternal mortality in high HIV prevalence regions. A higher increase in MMR trend during the period before implementation (2004–2006) and a relatively lower increase MMR trend after implementation of antenatal syphilis POC test exposure (2008–2014) was demonstrated. The increase in MMR trends before and after the exposure were significant.

To the best of our knowledge, this is the first study that has evaluated the impact of syphilis POC testing on MMR in a high HIV prevalence resource-limited setting. Our recent systematic review has shown a lack of evidence on the impact of syphilis POC diagnostics on maternal outcomes of HIV-infected patients [4]. A quasi-experimental interrupted time series design was employed to determine the impact of syphilis POC testing on maternal mortality ratio (MMR) in KZN. An interrupted time series is the most powerful quasi-experimental approach for evaluating effects of presence and absence of an exposure on outcomes [24,28]. This study design has enabled estimation of the change in MMR levels during the period of implementation, before and after implementation of syphilis POC test intervention, leading to determination of potential exposure effect on maternal mortality. This sharp change in the MMR trend marked the beginning of the second segment of the interrupted time series and does not reflect the immediate effect of discontinuation of syphilis POC testing intervention. Therefore, the interruption will occur at this data point (2007). The trend changes after this data point (2007) reflect the potential effect of introduction of syphilis POC testing in KZN. It is also worth noting the sharp drop after 2007 and a sharp rise in MMR in 2009, which was caused by missing data during 2008. The model used this data analysis included an omission command for the 2008 data points. Therefore the 2008 missing data was disregarding during analysis to ensure reliability of the model output.

DHIS data quality was a major limitation in this study [25]. Moreover, although syphilis infections have been associated with an increased risk of HIV transmission among pregnant women, the prevalence of syphilis is low in KZN. Therefore, in comparison to other disease conditions such as HIV, which have a high prevalence among women in KZN [29], the introduction of syphilis POC testing as a single exposure will not have a substantial impact on maternal mortality. However, due to the POC implementation dates (1998) for HIV and syphilis (2007) and the lack of archived DHIS MMR records prior to 2004, syphilis POC testing was the most suitable exposure for this study. During the analysis of monthly the MMR, data outliers which may have shifted the slope of the regression segments were detected. The sudden drop (34.2%) in MMR from 2007 to 2008 demonstrates inconsistencies in the data set. This finding is supported by a previous study which was aimed at introducing data improvement exposure for indicators in selected clinics in KZN in May 2008 [26]. This study revealed a significant improvement in data completeness from 26% before introduction of the exposure to 64% after the exposure, and also demonstrated a significant increase in data accuracy from 37% to 65% ($p < 0.0001$) after the exposure [26]. This was a retrospective study that used available routine DHIS data to answer the research question. The DHIS data did not contain the number of patients who were exposed to syphilis testing during each year. However, we are aware that all pregnant women are offered syphilis tests as part of routine antenatal test. Another limitation of this study is that our model only used DHIS data, which did not include data on pre-eclampsia cases. Pre-eclampsia is the leading cause of maternal and fetal morbidity and mortality worldwide [30–32]. It is a pregnancy-induced disorder reported to cause complications in approximately 5–7% of pregnancies.

The 2011 World Health Organization (WHO) global HIV/AIDS response has shown that up to one-third of the women attending antenatal care clinics are not tested for syphilis [33]. Maternal syphilis infections continue to affect large numbers of pregnant women, causing substantial perinatal morbidity and mortality that could be prevented by early testing and treatment [34,35]. The use of syphilis POC testing has been shown to result in health system strengthening and saving newborn lives [12]. Bearing in mind the reported increase in HIV-related maternal mortality in KZN [36] and the potential impact of syphilis POC testing on reducing MMR demonstrated in this study, there is a need for scaling up of syphilis POC testing. Although the results show the potential impact of syphilis POC testing on reducing maternal mortality, the level of MMR is still increasing. This demonstrates the need for additional interventions to deduce maternal mortality post-intervention.

As POC tests are being increasingly designed for use in resource-limited settings [37,38], rigorous assessment of the impact of current and future POC tests on key health outcomes is crucial in order to justify scale up or test replacement. This is supported by De Schacht et al. studies which recommend the need to identify optimal health delivery strategies to effectively bring the impact of technological advances such as POC testing to patients that are most at need [13]. Due to the recently reported increasing prevalence of HIV among women in KZN [29], detection of treatable infections that are associated with HIV transmission is crucial for the reduction of HIV-related maternal mortality. Future modelling studies on the impact of POC tests in KZN should exclude MMR data collected in 2008 to improve the reliability of the results.

5. Conclusions

The results of this study show an increasing maternal mortality ratio in KZN, South Africa. It also demonstrated the potential impact of antenatal syphilis POC test exposure on reducing the increase in MMR. However, the impact was in consideration of confounding factors related to MMR in these settings, thus the results require confirmation by use of a more rigorous study design. Bearing in mind the high importance of improving maternal outcomes in high HIV prevalent regions, efforts to help in the continual improvement of POC testing interventions aimed at improving maternal mortality are essential, particularly in these settings.

Supplementary Materials: Supplementary materials can be found at http://www.mdpi.com/2075-4418/9/4/218/s1. Table S1, Maternal deaths by year and month for all KZN.

Author Contributions: T.P.M.-T., B.S. and P.K.D. conceptualised and designed the study. T.P.M.-T. and B.S. carried out the analysis and produced the first draft of the manuscript. P.K.D. and D.K. commented on this draft and contributed to the final version. All authors read and approved the final manuscript.

Funding: This study is funded by the UKZN College of Health Sciences; South African Centre of Excellence for Epidemiology and Modelling Analysis (SACEMA), the African Population and Health Research Centre, and the National Institute of Allergy and Infectious Disease of the National Institutes of Health (K23 AI108293).

Acknowledgments: We would like to that the KwaZulu-Natal Department of Health, DHIS office for granting us access to data used for this study.

Conflicts of Interest: The authors declare no conflict of interest.

References

1. UNAIDS. The Gap Report. Available online: http://www.unaids.org/sites/default/files/media_asset/UNAIDS_Gap_report_en.pdf (accessed on 18 November 2019).
2. Department of Health. National Strategic Plan on HIV, STIs and TB 2012–2016. Available online: https://www.google.com.hk/url?sa=t&rct=j&q=&esrc=s&source=web&cd=3&ved=2ahUKEwiosYbwyZ3mAhXFGaYKHe2XBJEQFjACegQIBRAC&url=http%3A%2F%2Fwww.health.gov.za%2Findex.php%2Fshortcodes%2F2015-03-29-10-42-47%2F2015-04-30-08-18-10%2F2015-04-30-08-21-56%3Fdownload%3D579%3Ahiv-national-strategic-plan-on-hiv-stis-and-tb-2012-2016-summary&usg=AOvVaw2VI-h6VYlAzWt1sugeKjFt (accessed on 5 December 2019).
3. Statistics South Africa. Mid-year Population Estimates. Available online: http://www.statssa.gov.za/publications/P0302/P03022019.pdf (accessed on 3 November 2019).
4. Mashamba-Thompson, T.P.; Morgan, R.L.; Sartorius, B.; Dennis, B.; Drain, P.K.; Thabane, L. Effect of point-of-care diagnostics on maternal outcomes in human immunodeficiency virus–infected women: systematic review and meta-analysis. *Point Care* **2017**, *16*, 67. [CrossRef] [PubMed]
5. Amnesty International. Struggle for Maternal Health Barriers to Antenatal Care in South Africa; 2014. Available online: https://cisp.cachefly.net/assets/articles/attachments/51965_amnesty_southafrica530062014en.pdf (accessed on 5 December 2019).
6. Bronzan, R.N.; Mwesigwa-Kayongo, D.C.; Narkunas, D.; Schmid, G.P.; Neilsen, G.A.; Ballard, R.C.; Karuhije, P.; Ddamba, J.; Nombekela, E.; Hoyi, G. Onsite rapid antenatal syphilis screening with an immunochromatographic strip improves case detection and treatment in rural South African clinics. *Sex. Transm. Dis.* **2007**, *34*, S55–S60. [CrossRef] [PubMed]
7. Pronyk, P.; Kim, J.; Makhubele, M.; Hargreaves, J.; Mohlala, R.; Hausler, H. Introduction of voluntary counselling and rapid testing for HIV in rural South Africa: From theory to practice. *AIDS Care* **2002**, *14*, 859–865. [CrossRef] [PubMed]
8. Dhatt, R.; Theobald, S.; Buzuzi, S.; Ros, B.; Vong, S.; Muraya, K.; Molyneux, S.; Hawkins, K.; González-Beiras, C.; Ronsin, K. The role of women's leadership and gender equity in leadership and health system strengthening. *Glob. HealthEpidemiol. Genom.* **2017**, *2*. [CrossRef] [PubMed]
9. Mullick, S.; Beksinksa, M.; Msomi, S. Treatment for syphilis in antenatal care: Compliance with the three dose standard treatment regimen. *Sex. Transm. Infect.* **2005**, *81*, 220–222. [CrossRef] [PubMed]
10. Kuupiel, D.; Tlou, B.; Bawontuo, V.; Mashamba-Thompson, T.P. Accessibility of pregnancy-related point-of-care diagnostic tests for maternal healthcare in rural primary healthcare facilities in Northern Ghana: A cross-sectional survey. *Heliyon* **2019**, *5*, e01236. [CrossRef]
11. Kuupiel, D.; Adu, K.M.; Bawontuo, V.; Mashamba-Thompson, T.P. Geographical Accessibility to District Hospitals/Medical Laboratories for Comprehensive Antenatal Point-of-Care Diagnostic Services in the Upper East Region, Ghana. *EClinicalMedicine* **2019**, *13*, 74–80. [CrossRef]
12. Mabey, D.C.; Sollis, K.A.; Kelly, H.A.; Benzaken, A.S.; Bitarakwate, E.; Changalucha, J.; Chen, X.-S.; Yin, Y.-P.; Garcia, P.J.; Strasser, S. Point-of-care tests to strengthen health systems and save newborn lives: The case of syphilis. *PLoS Med.* **2012**, *9*, e1001233. [CrossRef]
13. De Schacht, C.; Lucas, C.; Sitoe, N.; Machekano, R.; Chongo, P.; Temmerman, M.; Tobaiwa, O.; Guay, L.; Kassaye, S.; Jani, I.V. Implementation of point-of-care diagnostics leads to variable uptake of syphilis, anemia and CD4+ T-Cell count testing in rural maternal and child health clinics. *PLoS ONE* **2015**, *10*, e0135744. [CrossRef]
14. Mashamba-Thompson, T.; Sartorius, B.; Drain, P. Operational assessment of point-of-care diagnostics in rural primary healthcare clinics of KwaZulu-Natal, South Africa: A cross-sectional survey. *BMC Health Serv. Res.* **2018**, *18*, 380. [CrossRef]
15. Lynn, W.; Lightman, S. Syphilis and HIV: A dangerous combination. *Lancet Infect. Dis.* **2004**, *4*, 456–466. [CrossRef]

16. Berman, S.M. Maternal syphilis: Pathophysiology and treatment. *Bull. World Health Organ.* **2004**, *82*, 433–438. [PubMed]
17. Blencowe, H.; Cousens, S.; Kamb, M.; Berman, S.; Lawn, J.E. Lives Saved Tool supplement detection and treatment of syphilis in pregnancy to reduce syphilis related stillbirths and neonatal mortality. *BMC Public Health* **2011**, *11*, S9. [CrossRef] [PubMed]
18. Hawkes, S.; Matin, N.; Broutet, N.; Low, N. Effectiveness of interventions to improve screening for syphilis in pregnancy: A systematic review and meta-analysis. *Lancet Infect. Dis.* **2011**, *11*, 684–691. [CrossRef]
19. Buchacz, K.; Patel, P.; Taylor, M.; Kerndt, P.R.; Byers, R.H.; Holmberg, S.D.; Klausner, J.D. Syphilis increases HIV viral load and decreases CD4 cell counts in HIV-infected patients with new syphilis infections. *Aids* **2004**, *18*, 2075–2079. [CrossRef] [PubMed]
20. Yeganeh, N.; Watts, H.D.; Camarca, M.; Soares, G.; Joao, E.; Pilotto, J.H.; Gray, G.; Theron, G.; Santos, B.; Fonseca, R. Syphilis in HIV-infected Mothers and Infants: Results from the NICHD/HPTN 040 Study. *Pediatric Infect. Dis. J.* **2015**, *34*, e52–e57. [CrossRef]
21. Khan, M.; Pillay, T.; Moodley, J.M.; Connolly, C.A.; Durban Perinatal TB HIV-1 Study Group. Maternal mortality associated with tuberculosis–HIV-1 co-infection in Durban, South Africa. *Aids* **2001**, *15*, 1857–1863. [CrossRef]
22. Mashamba-Thompson, T.; Drain, P.; Sartorius, B. Evaluating the accessibility and utility of HIV-related point-of-care diagnostics for maternal health in rural South Africa: A study protocol. *BMJ Open* **2016**, *6*, e011155. [CrossRef]
23. Shadish, W.R.; Cook, T.D.; Campbell, D.T. Experimental and quasi-experimental designs for generalized causal inference. *J. Am. Stat. Assoc.* **2005**, *100*, 708.
24. Taljaard, M.; McKenzie, J.E.; Ramsay, C.R.; Grimshaw, J.M. The use of segmented regression in analysing interrupted time series studies: An example in pre-hospital ambulance care. *Implement. Sci.* **2014**, *9*, 77. [CrossRef]
25. Mate, K.S.; Bennett, B.; Mphatswe, W.; Barker, P.; Rollins, N. Challenges for routine health system data management in a large public programme to prevent mother-to-child HIV transmission in South Africa. *PLoS ONE* **2009**, *4*, e5483. [CrossRef] [PubMed]
26. Mphatswe, W.; Mate, K.S.; Bennett, B.; Ngidi, H.; Reddy, J.; Barker, P.M.; Rollins, N. Improving public health information: A data quality intervention in KwaZulu-Natal, South Africa. *Bull. World Health Organ.* **2012**, *90*, 176–182. [CrossRef] [PubMed]
27. Wagner, A.; Soumerai, S.; Zhang, F.; Ross-Degnan, D. Segmented regression analysis of interrupted time series studies in medication use research. *J. Clin. Pharm. Ther.* **2002**, *27*, 299–309. [CrossRef] [PubMed]
28. Campbell, D.T.; Stanley, J.C. Experimental and Quasi-Experimental Designs for Research; Ravenio Books: 2015. Available online: https://apps.who.int/iris/bitstream/handle/10665/44787/9789241502986_eng.pdf (accessed on 5 December 2019).
29. Kharsany, A.B.; Frohlich, J.A.; Yende-Zuma, N.; Mahlase, G.; Samsunder, N.; Dellar, R.C.; Zuma-Mkhonza, M.; Karim, S.S.A.; Karim, Q.A. Trends in HIV prevalence in pregnant women in rural South Africa. *Jaids J. Acquir. Immune Defic. Syndr.* **2015**, *70*, 289–295. [CrossRef]
30. Lagana, A.S.; Vitale, S.G.; Sapia, F.; Valenti, G.; Corrado, F.; Padula, F.; Rapisarda, A.M.C.; D'Anna, R. miRNA expression for early diagnosis of preeclampsia onset: Hope or hype? *J. Matern.-Fetal Neonatal Med.* **2018**, *31*, 817–821. [CrossRef]
31. Laganà, A.S.; Giordano, D.; Loddo, S.; Zoccali, G.; Vitale, S.G.; Santamaria, A.; Buemi, M.; D'Anna, R. Decreased Endothelial Progenitor Cells (EPCs) and increased Natural Killer (NK) cells in peripheral blood as possible early markers of preeclampsia: A case-control analysis. *Arch. Gynecol. Obstet.* **2017**, *295*, 867–872. [CrossRef]
32. Salman, H.; Shah, M.; Ali, A.; Aziz, A.; Vitale, S.G. Assessment of Relationship of Serum Neurokinin-B Level in the Pathophysiology of Pre-eclampsia: A Case–Control Study. *Adv. Ther.* **2018**, *35*, 1114–1121. [CrossRef]
33. WHO; UNAiDS; Unicef. Global HIV/AIDS Response: Epidemic Update and Health Sector Progress Towards Universal Access: Progress Report 2011. Available online: https://scholar.google.com.hk/scholar?hl=zh-CN&as_sdt=0%2C5&q=34.%09WHo%2C+UNAiDS%2C+Unicef.+Global+HIV%2FAIDS+response%3A+Epidemic+update+and+health+sector+progress+towards+universal+access%3A+Progress+report+2011.&btnG=#d=gs_cit&u=%2Fscholar%3Fq%3Dinfo%3As_Alx9YRhYMJ%3Ascholar.google.com%2F%26output%3Dcite%26scirp%3D0%26hl%3Dzh-CN (accessed on 10 December 2019).

34. Newman, L.; Kamb, M.; Hawkes, S.; Gomez, G.; Say, L.; Seuc, A.; Broutet, N. Global estimates of syphilis in pregnancy and associated adverse outcomes: Analysis of multinational antenatal surveillance data. *PLoS Med.* **2013**, *10*, e1001396. [CrossRef]
35. Moline, H.R.; Smith, J.F., Jr. The continuing threat of syphilis in pregnancy. *Curr. Opin. Obstet. Gynecol.* **2016**, *28*, 101–104. [CrossRef]
36. Lebastchi, A.H.; Yuh, D.D. Nationwide survey of US integrated 6-year cardiothoracic surgical residents. *J. Thorac. Cardiovasc. Surg.* **2014**, *148*, 401–407. [CrossRef] [PubMed]
37. Drain, P.K.; Hyle, E.P.; Noubary, F.; Freedberg, K.A.; Wilson, D.; Bishai, W.R.; Rodriguez, W.; Bassett, I.V. Diagnostic point-of-care tests in resource-limited settings. *Lancet Infect. Dis.* **2014**, *14*, 239–249. [CrossRef]
38. Mabey, D.; Peeling, R.W.; Ustianowski, A.; Perkins, M.D. Diagnostics for the developing world. *Nat. Rev. Microbiol.* **2004**, *2*, 231–240. [CrossRef] [PubMed]

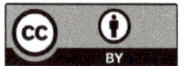 © 2019 by the authors. Licensee MDPI, Basel, Switzerland. This article is an open access article distributed under the terms and conditions of the Creative Commons Attribution (CC BY) license (http://creativecommons.org/licenses/by/4.0/).

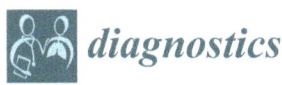

Article

Geographical Accessibility to Glucose-6-Phosphate Dioxygenase Deficiency Point-of-Care Testing for Antenatal Care in Ghana

Desmond Kuupiel [1,2,*], Kwame M. Adu [3], Vitalis Bawontuo [2,4], Duncan A. Adogboba [5], Paul K. Drain [6], Mosa Moshabela [1] and Tivani P. Mashamba-Thompson [1,7]

[1] Department of Public Health Medicine, School of Nursing and Public Health, University of KwaZulu-Natal, Durban 4041, South Africa; Moshabela@ukzn.ac.za (M.M.); Mashamba-Thompson@ukzn.ac.za (T.P.M.-T.)
[2] Research for Sustainable Development Consult, Sunyani, Ghana; bawontuovitalis@yahoo.com
[3] Department of Geography, University of Ghana, Legon, Ghana; meous007@gmail.com
[4] Faculty of Health and Allied Sciences, Catholic University College of Ghana, Fiapre, Sunyani, Ghana
[5] Regional Health Directorate, Ghana Health Service, Upper East Region, Bolgatanga, Ghana; alemna@gmail.com
[6] Department of Global Health, University of Washington, Seattle, WA 98195, USA; pkdrain@uw.edu
[7] Department of Public Health, Faculty of Health Sciences, University of Limpopo, Polokwane 0723, South Africa
* Correspondence: desmondkuupiel98@hotmail.com; Tel.: +27-73-556-8200 or +23-355-097-2968

Received: 10 March 2020; Accepted: 8 April 2020; Published: 16 April 2020

Abstract: Background: Glucose-6-Phosphate Dehydrogenase (G6PD) deficiency screening test is essential for malaria treatment, control, and elimination programs. G6PD deficient individuals are at high risk of severe hemolysis when given anti-malarial drugs such as primaquine, quinine, other sulphonamide-containing medicines, and chloroquine, which has recently been shown to be potent for the treatment of coronavirus disease (COVID-19). We evaluated the geographical accessibility to POC testing for G6PD deficiency in Ghana, a malaria-endemic country. Methods: We obtained the geographic information of 100 randomly sampled clinics previously included in a cross-sectional survey. We also obtained the geolocated data of all public hospitals providing G6PD deficiency testing services in the region. Using ArcGIS 10.5, we quantified geographical access to G6PD deficiency screening test and identified clinics as well as visualize locations with poor access for targeted improvement. The travel time was estimated using an assumed speed of 20 km per hour. Findings: Of the 100 clinics, 58% were Community-based Health Planning and Services facilities, and 42% were sub-district health centers. The majority (92%) were Ghana Health Service facilities, and the remaining 8% were Christian Health Association of Ghana facilities. Access to G6PD deficiency screening test was varied across the districts, and G6PD deficiency screening test was available in all eight public hospitals. This implies that the health facility-to-population ratio for G6PD deficiency testing service was approximately 1:159,210 (8/1,273,677) population. The spatial analysis quantified the current mean distance to a G6PD deficiency testing service from all locations in the region to be 34 ± 14 km, and travel time (68 ± 27 min). The estimated mean distance from a clinic to a district hospital for G6PD deficiency testing services was 15 ± 11 km, and travel time (46 ± 33 min). Conclusion: Access to POC testing for G6PD deficiency in Ghana was poor. Given the challenges associated with G6PD deficiency, it would be essential to improve access to G6PD deficiency POC testing to facilitate administration of sulphadoxine-pyrimethamine to pregnant women, full implementation of the malaria control program in Ghana, and treatment of COVID-19 patients with chloroquine in malaria-endemic countries. To enable the World Health Organization include appropriate G6PD POC diagnostic tests in its list of essential in-vitro diagnostics for use in resource-limited settings, we recommend a wider evaluation of available POC diagnostic tests for G6PD deficiency, particularly in malaria-endemic countries.

Keywords: geographical access; glucose-6-phosphate dioxygenase deficiency; point-of-care testing; antenatal care; upper east region; Ghana

---

1. Introduction

Glucose-6-phosphate dehydrogenase (G6PD) deficiency is a sex-link hereditary mutation on the X-chromosome [1–3]. G6PD is an enzyme that helps protect red blood cells from damage and premature destruction [2,3]. Although most G6PD deficiency patients do not show clinical signs and symptoms, it is commonly characterized by abnormally low levels of G6PD, and some variants could be fatal due to complete loss of enzyme activity [2,3]. Globally, G6PD deficiency affects approximately 400 million people and its prevalence is highest particularly, in malaria-endemic countries ranging from 5 to 24% [4,5]. A systematic review in 2009 showed that Sub-Saharan African (SSA) countries accounted for the highest G6PD prevalence before and after adjusting for the assessment method [4]. The meta-analysis also showed a high degree of geographical heterogeneity of G6PD prevalence estimates, which seemed to be due to differences in G6PD deficiency assessment and diagnostic procedures [4]. The magnitude and geographical (global, regional, and country-level) heterogeneity of G6PD deficiency prevalence rates have public health implications, especially in malaria control or elimination programs involving the administration of antimalarial medicines for most malaria-endemic countries such as Ghana. G6PD deficient individuals are at high risk of severe hemolysis when given anti-malarial drugs such as primaquine, quinine, other sulphonamide-containing medicines [6–8], and chloroquine which has been shown to be potent for the treatment of coronavirus disease (COVID-19) [6,9,10], These drugs may cause an irreversible oxidative activity of the body's metabolites on erythrocytes [7,8].

Ghana is at risk of malaria throughout the year with over 21% of malaria parasitemia of which approximately 98% result from Plasmodium falciparum infection [11,12]. Ghana is ranked fourth alongside Burkina Faso, Uganda, and accounted for 4% of the world's 219 million malaria cases in 2017 according to a World Health Organization (WHO) 2018 report [13,14]. Malaria infection during pregnancy has substantial risk for the mother, her fetus and the newborn such as placental malaria infection, low birth weight, and severe maternal anemia [15–20]. As part of the intermittent preventive treatment during pregnancy (IPTp) in Ghana, a single of sulphadoxine-pyrimethamine (SP) is administered to pregnant women at predefined intervals after quickening (16 gestational weeks) to reduce malaria parasitemia and poor pregnancy outcomes as recommended by the WHO [15,21,22]. Although a low dose of SP has been reported to be highly effective in preventing malaria in pregnancy and reducing the consequences of malaria infection such as reduce placental malaria infection, reduction of low birth weight and severe maternal anemia [15–20], it contains sulphonamide, one of the groups of oxidant drugs capable of inducing hemolysis [2,3,23,24].

To address this, the anti-malaria drug policy for Ghana recommends that pregnant women be screened for G6PD deficiency and those with G6PD deficiency be excluded from IPTp with SP administration [22,25]. G6PD deficiency prevalence in Ghana has been estimated to range from 6.5 to 19% [26–28]. In view of this, it a policy of the Ghanaian Ministry of Health that the G6PD deficiency status of every pregnant woman should be checked during the first antenatal visit. However, G6PD deficiency testing in Ghana is still a laboratory-based test (microscopy) and may not be accessible to all pregnant women particularly, those accessing ANC in rural primary healthcare (PHC) clinics. Although previous studies assessed the availability and supply chain management of point-of-care (POC) test including G6PD deficiency tests [29–31], geographical accessibility to comprehensive ANC POC testing [32], and evaluated a POC testing device for G6PD deficiency [5], to date, no study in Ghana has assessed the geographical accessibility to POC testing for G6PD deficiency. To inform national policy on G6PD deficiency screening test, support treatment decisions with anti-malarial medicines and SP administration to pregnant women in rural PHC clinics, the national malaria control or elimination program, and to improve equity to healthcare, we mapped the geographical access (distance and travel time) to POC testing for G6PD deficiency using geographical information systems.

2. Methods

2.1. Study Design and Setting

This is a follow-up study on a prior cross-sectional study conducted to assess the accessibility of pregnancy-related POC diagnostic tests in the upper east region (UER) of Ghana [29]. Of the 100 participated PHC clinics in the earlier study, none was providing G6PD deficiency testing services in the region [29]. This current study, therefore, mapped the geographical access to POC testing for G6PD deficiency as part of ANC services. The study setting has been adequately described in the earlier published cross-sectional survey and audit [29,30]. The 2019 project population of the region is approximately 1,273,677 (51.6% females) and is considered largely (79%) rural and scattered in dispersed settlements [33].

2.2. Data Collection

We previously collected data on 100 randomly selected PHC clinics from all the districts in the UER as explained in the published cross-sectional survey [29]. We also collected data on all health facilities (district hospitals) providing G6PD deficiency testing in the region. To map the geographic access to G6PD deficiency testing services in UER, the geo-located data of the health facilities providing G6PD deficiency testing and that of PHC clinics were obtained from the Regional Health Directorate, and the use of global positioning system. Topographical data such as roads, rivers, and digital elevation models were obtained and juxtaposed with data obtained from the University of Ghana Remote Sensing and Geographic Information Systems laboratory to validate data accuracy. To allow for the results of spatial processes in a chosen unit of 'meters', the world geodetic system zone 30° N coordinate system was applied to all spatial data. PHC clinic information such as clinic type, ownership, availability of G6PD deficiency testing services, and name of nearest district hospital providing G6PD POC testing and location were obtained from the clinic managers using a questionnaire. The health facilities mentioned as accessed points were cross-checked to be sure of the availability of the G6PD deficiency testing service.

2.3. Variables and Operational Definitions

2.3.1. Availability

The availability of health facilities providing G6PD deficiency testing services.

2.3.2. Distance

The proximity from a PHC clinic/population to the nearest district hospital providing G6PD deficiency testing at point-of-care.

2.3.3. Travel Time

Estimated time likely to be spent by a patient or pregnant woman traveling from a PHC clinic or any location in UER to the entrance of a district hospital for a G6PD deficiency screening test.

2.4. Data Analysis and Mapping

We linked the data on PHC clinics, health facilities providing G6PD deficiency screening test, area, and the geographic coordinates of the health facilities to ArcGIS 10.4 software and a base map. All 100 PHC clinics from the earlier cross-sectional survey were used as inputs to quantify the distance in kilometers (km) to their nearest health facilities providing a G6PD deficiency screening test in the study area. The euclidean distance from the PHC clinic as well as from all areas of UER to the nearest health facility was calculated using the near function analysis tools in ArcGIS 10.5. We used an assumed speed of 20 km per hour of the most available and generally utilized public transport in the region known as "motor king" (a motorized tricycle) to estimate the travel time from all areas. The model and technique used to guesstimate the travel time from all locations in UER to the closest health facilities providing G6PD deficiency screening test in this current study are published in our previous studies [32,34]. The estimated distances and travel times for each of the Districts to the nearest health facility providing G6PD deficiency testing services from PHC clinics and all locations in the UER were exported to Stata V 14.0 software for analysis and the mean and standard deviation calculated and reported. A study showed that access to healthcare beyond 10 km has an association with higher risks of poor health outcomes [35]. Therefore, this current study considered location less ≤10 km to the nearest district hospital providing G6PD deficiency screening test as zones with good geographical access.

2.5. Ethics Approval

This study was approved by the Navrongo Health Research Centre Institutional Review Board/Ghana Health Service (approval number: NHRCIRB291) on 8th January 2018 and the University of KwaZulu-Natal Biomedical Research Ethics Committee (approval number: BE565/17) on 12 February 2018.

3. Results

3.1. Characteristics of the Participated PHC Clinics in the Study

One hundred PHC clinics were included in this study comprising of 58% Community-based Health Planning and Services (CHPS) facilities, and 42 sub-district health centers. Of the 100 participated PHC clinics, the majority (92%) were Ghana Health Service (GHS) facilities, and the remaining 8% were Christian Health Association of Ghana (CHAG) facilities.

3.2. Geographical Distribution of Public Health Facilities Providing G6PD Deficiency Testing in UER

POC testing for G6PD deficiency was available in all eight hospitals. This implies that the health facility-to-population ratio for G6PD deficiency POC testing in UER was approximately 1:159,210 (8/1,273,677) population, whilst the health facility-to-women of reproductive age (WORA) was about 1:38,210 (8/305683). Of these eight hospitals, six (6) were District Hospitals owned and managed by the GHS, one (1) owned by a Church (a member of the CHAG), and one (1) Regional Hospital. Of the thirteen administrative districts in the region, five districts (Binduri, Nabdam, Garu-Tempane, Pusiga, and Builsa South) had no health facility providing G6PD deficiency POC testing, as shown in Figure 1.

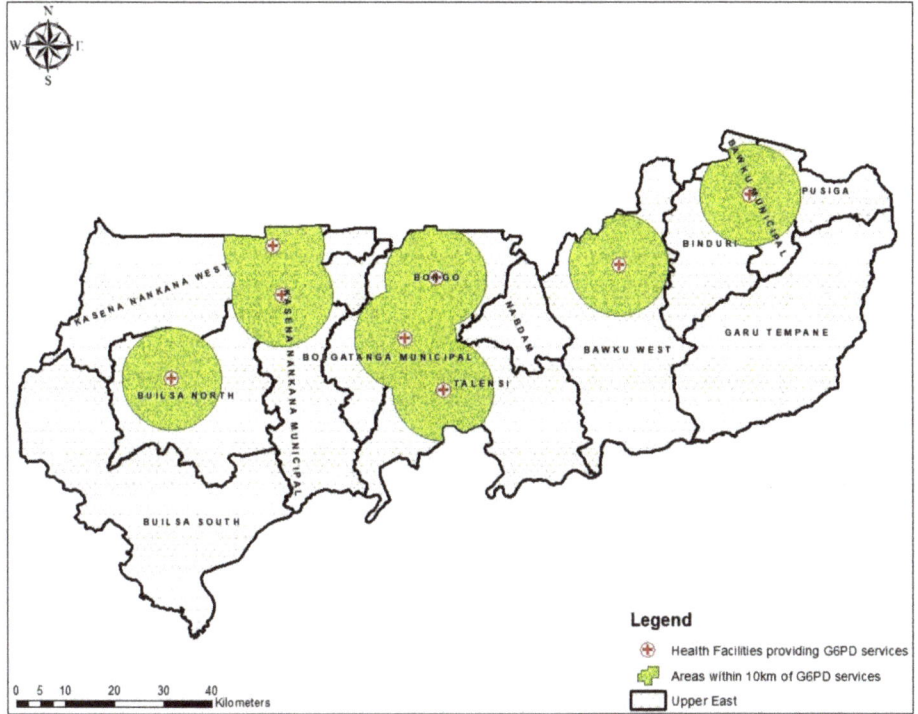

Figure 1. Map showing the geographic distribution of health facilities providing Glucose-6-Phosphate Dehydrogenase (G6PD) deficiency screening test and sites within 10 km distance from the health facility.

3.3. Geographical Access to Health Facilities for G6PD Deficiency POC Testing in the UER

We mapped the 100 randomly selected PHC clinics to the nearest hospital in the region providing G6PD deficiency testing and estimated the distance and travel time. Of the 100 PHC clinics, the majority (52%) were located in areas greater than 10 km to the nearest health facility where G6PD deficiency screening test. None of the participated clinics in three districts (Garu-Tempane, Nabdam, and Builsa South) was within 10 km proximity to the nearest health facility providing a G6PD deficiency screening test (Figure 2). The estimated mean distance from a PHC clinic to a hospital for G6PD deficiency screening test in the region was 15 ± 11 km, and the mean travel time was 46 ± 33 min based on a motorized tricycle speed of 20 km per hour.

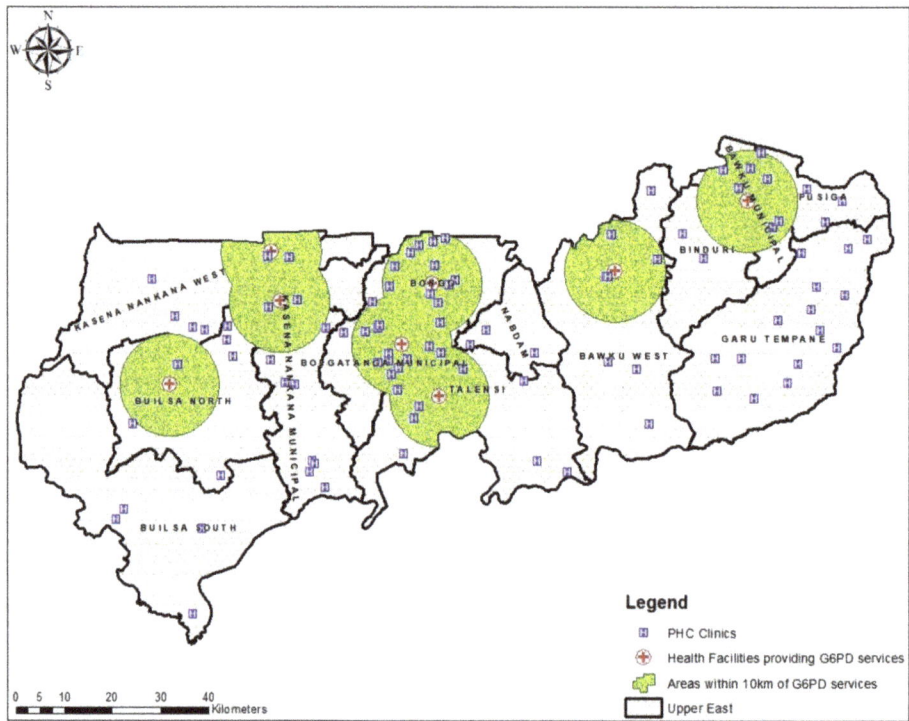

Figure 2. Map showing the distribution of the primary healthcare (PHC) clinics and distance within 10 km from the nearest health facility providing G6PD screening test.

Based on the 100 PHC clinics involved in this study, 3 districts (Bawku Municipal, Bolgatanga Municipal, and Bongo District) out of the 13 in the region recorded good geographical access (mean distance less than 10 km) to POC testing for G6PD deficiency in the region. Of the remaining ten districts that recorded poor geographical access to POC testing for G6PD deficiency, PHC clinics in the Builsa South and Garu-Tempane districts with mean distances of 30 ± 9 km (travel time; 89.6 ± 27.5 min) and 28 ± 6 km (travel time; 85 ± 18 min) respectively were shown to have poorer geographical access compared to the other districts.

We also quantified the distance and travel time from all locations in the region to the closest health facility for G6PD deficiency screening test. The results show varied geographical access to POC testing for G6PD deficiency in all 13 districts. The results show populations in the Bolgatanga Municipality has better access to health facilities for G6PD deficiency testing [mean distance = 23 km; SD = 9, mean travel time = 46 min; SD = 19] whilst Garu-Tempane District recorded the poorest [mean distance = 50 km; SD = 17, mean travel time = 99 min; SD = 34]. The mean distance and traveling time using all locations were 34 ± 14 km and 68 ± 26 min respectively. Figures 3 and 4 respectively present the mean distance and travel time to POC testing for G6PD deficiency per district in the region.

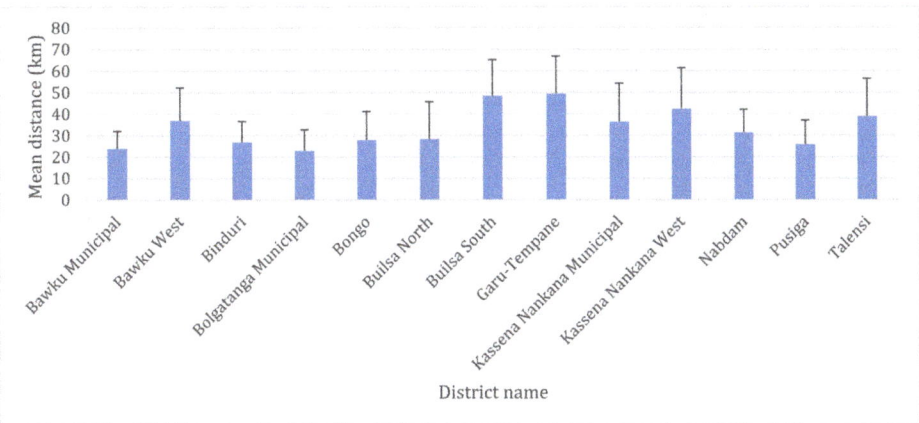

Figure 3. Mean distance and standard deviation from all locations to the nearest hospital providing G6PD deficiency point-of-care (POC) testing services in the upper east region (UER) by districts.

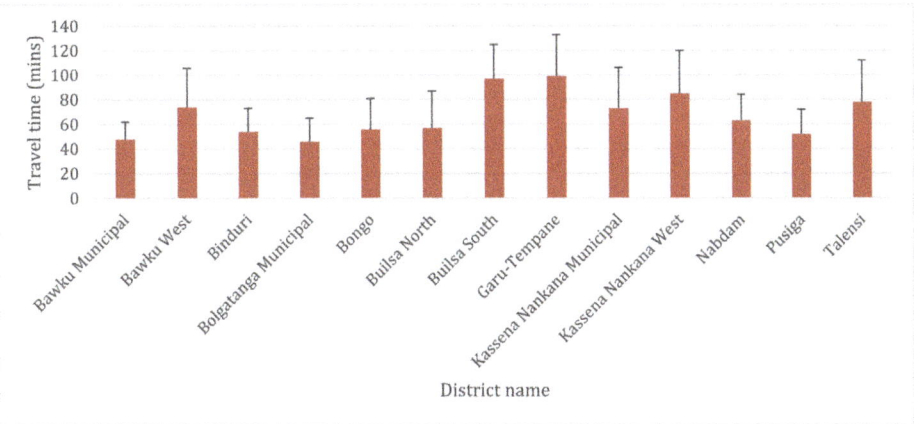

Figure 4. Mean travel time and standard deviation from all locations to the nearest hospital providing G6PD deficiency POC testing services in the UER by districts.

4. Discussion

This study revealed limited availability of health facilities offering G6PD deficiency screening test in the region. All PHC clinics lacked a POC device for G6PD deficiency screening. G6PD deficiency screening test was available in districts where a hospital was present and providing laboratory services. Moreover, the geographical access to POC testing for G6PD deficiency in the region was poor and varied across the districts.

Similarly to the present study findings, Adu-Gyasi and colleagues' 2015 study in Ghana aimed to evaluate a G6PD deficiency POC device revealed limited availability of health facilities providing G6PD deficiency screening test [5]. Their study evidenced that no health facility except the research institution was providing G6PD deficiency screening as an essential healthcare service in their study area [5]. Elsewhere, Therrell and colleagues in 2015 reported that despite the highest prevalence of G6PD deficiency in Africa and the Middle East, these regions have the poorest access to G6PD deficiency screening tests [36]. Anderle and colleagues in their review also observed that G6PD deficiency screening services are mostly accessible to urban populations close to health facilities that provide the service [37]. Contrary to the current study findings, Ley and colleagues' study in 2015 evidenced the availability of G6PD deficiency microscopy screening and rapid diagnostic testing (RDTs) services at all health facilities as well as community-level health facilities in Bangladesh [38]. Ley and colleagues further evinced the availability of G6PD deficiency microscopy screening and RDTs service in all hospital and clinics, and the availability of RDTs only at community-level health facilities in Cambodia [38]. Ley and colleagues study additionally showed that in the Philippines, G6PD deficiency microscopy screening was found to be available in hospitals as well as municipal health clinics [38]. Moreover, access to G6PD deficiency screening service was described to be high in the Asia Pacific region where about six countries were reported to be providing the service to the general population and sub-populations such as newborns [36].

Although we found no study reporting on the geographical access to POC testing for G6PD deficiency either in Ghana or elsewhere, previous studies that assessed the geographical access to health facilities for comprehensive ANC service, and tuberculosis POC testing in UER reported similarly poor accessibility with district variation as well as random spatial distribution of the health facilities providing the services [32,34,39]. The poor geographical accessibility to POC testing for G6PD deficiency evidenced by this current study has potential implications on Ghana's malaria control program, screening of pregnant women prior to SP administration, and screening of newborns for G6PD deficiency as recommended by the WHO. Healthcare providers in rural PHC clinics mostly likely may be prescribing anti-malarial drugs to patients without knowledge of their G6PD deficiency status. It is also possible pregnant women particularly primigravidas (first timers) receiving ANC services in rural PHC clinics whose G6PD deficiency statuses were previously unknown may be denied SP administration unjustifiably. Traveling long distances to access G6PD deficiency screening test have financial implications, long waiting time for test results, and may result in patient dissatisfaction. Hence, patients or pregnant women may fail to go for a G6PD screening test at the referral hospital and this consequently may affect both maternal and newborn health outcomes.

To address disparities with regards to access to G6PD deficiency testing services, inform rural healthcare providers decisions on SP or anti-malarial therapy, and improve malaria, maternal, and newborn health outcomes, we recommend the implementation of G6PD POC testing at rural PHC clinics in Ghana. For instance, locations in UER with poor geographical access to G6PD deficiency testing services as visualized in Figure 5 should be prioritized for improvement. Although the WHO has not included a G6PD deficiency screening test as one of the tests to be performed in PHC clinics in the essential list of in vitro diagnostics, several G6PD deficiency POC testing devices and RDTs are available in recent time and are have been used in countries such as Bangladesh and Cambodia [38] to improve access to G6PD deficiency testing service. Implementation of appropriate POC diagnostic tests for G6PD deficiency testing in rural and resource-limited health facilities in Ghana and other malaria-endemic countries with poor access to G6PD deficiency testing can help resolve the dilemma with the administration of SP and other antimalarial medicines health providers in those areas experience. It will also reduce the potential catastrophic indirect cost associated with accessing the service such as transportation cost, loss of man-hours at hospitals, and other unforeseen risks resulting from traveling long distances with poor transportation systems.

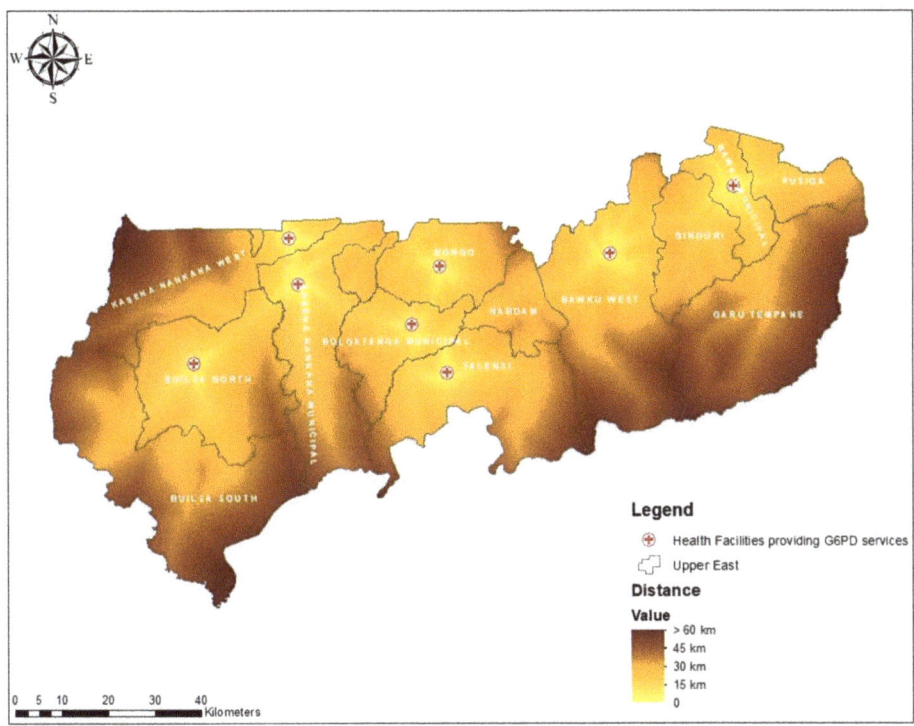

Figure 5. Map showing the distribution of distance (km) from all residential areas to health facilities providing G6PD screening test in the UER.

An additional benefit for implementing POC testing for G6PD deficiency at rural PHC clinics in UER will be a reduction of traveling time from all areas (Figure 6) and improve accessibility to the service. This may lead to increase utilization of the service and improve health outcomes. Furthermore, implementing G6PD deficiency screening tests at PHC clinics will help improve Ghana's malaria control program as well as contribute to Ghana's quest to attain universal health coverage. Moreover, the ability of health providers in resource-limited settings to test the G6PD deficiency status of pregnant women potentially can help them report promptly hemolytic anemia cases caused by G6PD deficiency may during pregnancy management to prevent hematological and several possible serious obstetrical complications such as fetus malformations, infertility, bilirubin-induced neurological damage in newborns, and death [6,40]. In view of these, we recommend a wider implementation of appropriate diagnostic tests for G6PD deficiency testing in rural and resource-limited settings health facilities to improve G6PD deficiency status testing of pregnant women and patients prior to the administration of SP and other antimalaria medicines as well as, facilitate the malaria control/elimination programs with primaquine in malaria-endemic countries.

Moreover, chloroquine has recently been shown to be a useful drug for the treatment of Coronavirus Disease 2019 (COVID-19) [10]. which has so far infected over 1,200,000 million people with more than 62,000 deaths [41]. Based on this, some countries are considering the use of chloroquine to treat COVID-19 cases, despite the safety concerns raised regarding its use due to the possibility of chloroquine causing hemolysis in patients with G6PD deficiency [9]. Considering this, checking the G6PD deficiency status of a COVID-19 patient prior to treatment with chloroquine may be ideal, particularly in malaria-endemic countries such as Ghana. Hence, it would be prudent to improve the availability of and accessibility to POC testing for G6PD deficiency prior to the recommendation of the use of chloroquine for treatment of COVID-19 patients in malaria-endemic countries such as Ghana.

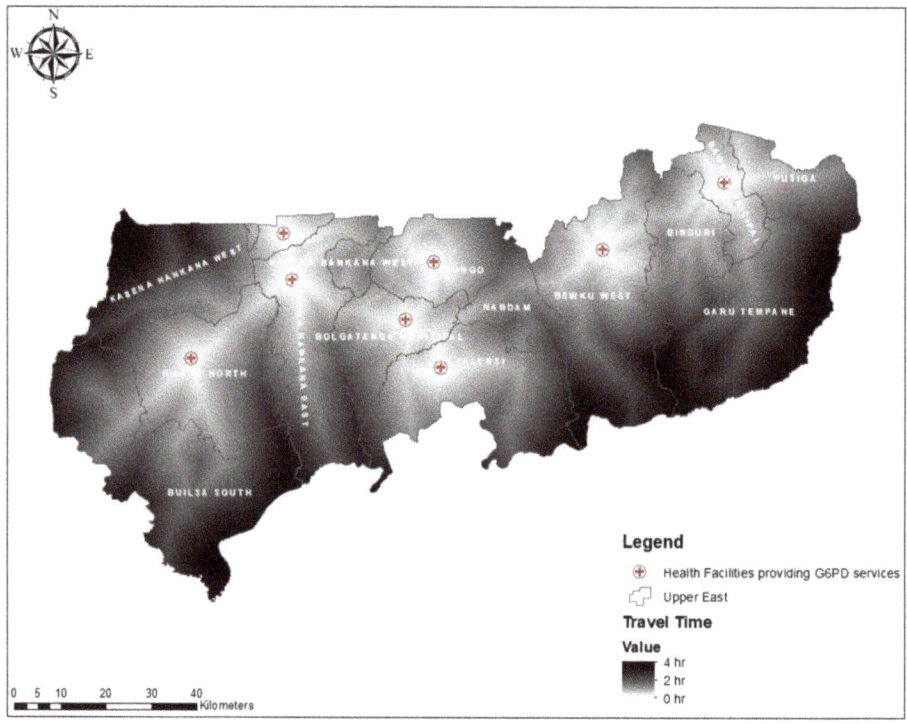

Figure 6. Map showing the distribution of travel time (mins) from all residential areas to health facilities providing G6PD screening test in the UER.

Using GIS to inform the implementation of health services has been shown to be useful [42–44]. GIS effectively enables the implementation of POC testing in health networks to streamline decision making at the POC [45]. Geospatial science has also been proven to be useful in creating solutions for population access to POC testing during emergencies, outbreaks, and disasters such as the present COVID-19 pandemic [46]. Hence, GIS helps improve patient outcomes, time and money, ensure that the health networks are sufficiently resourced to deliver needed health services to the population [45]. Despite these strengths, there are several limitations worth noting such as our inability to include non-spatial factors in the analysis. Non-spatial factors such as the income of a patient [47], age, cultural practices, education, and others can also influence the utilization of a health service even if the service is very close to the individual [48]. Although this study is recommending implementation of POC testing for G6PD deficiency at rural PHC clinics, it did not assess the cost-benefit analysis of its implementation. However, knowing the G6PD status of a patient is useful clinical information and the cost of implementing POC for G6PD deficiency testing service at rural PHC clinics by the Government of Ghana should not be a reason to deny a special sub-population such as pregnant women and newborns access to G6PD deficiency testing because Ghana is a malaria-endemic country. It is also possible some private hospitals and medical laboratories within the region may be providing G6PD deficiency screening test and where not included in this study's analysis. The travel time estimation provided by this study was dependent on only one mode of public transport using an assumed speed which might be inaccurate. Moreover, this study was only limited to only one region in Ghana and therefore the findings may not necessarily apply to the remaining fifteen regions in the country. We, therefore, recommend future researches to focus on areas such as the non-spatial factors, cost-benefit analysis of implementing POC testing for G6PD deficiency at PHC clinics not captured by this study. We also recommend a similar study in the other fifteen regions of Ghana. We further recommend future studies to included other modes of transportation such as walking, car, motorbike, bicycle, and others where applicable in the analysis. Nonetheless, this study has provided evidence-based information useful for policy decision making for targeted improvement of POC testing for G6PD deficiency in the UER. This study also provides baseline information for future studies since it is the first study to evaluate the geographical accessibility to POC testing for G6PD deficiency in Ghana and perhaps, worldwide.

5. Conclusions

G6PD deficiency POC test permits clinical diagnostic decisions either to administer anti-malarial drugs/SP or not in resource-limited settings and useful for improving health outcomes and the cost of accessing G6PD testing services. Spatial analysis estimated current mean distance and travel to a G6PD deficiency testing center from all locations in UER to be over 33 km and 60 min respectively using a motorized tricycle. This could be reduced significantly with the implementation of POC testing for G6PD deficiency at PHC clinics located more than 10 km away from a health facility. Given the challenges associated with G6PD deficiency, it would be essential to improve access to G6PD deficiency POC testing to facilitate administration of sulphadoxine-pyrimethamine to pregnant women, full implementation of the malaria control program in Ghana, and treatment of COVID-19 patients with chloroquine in malaria-endemic countries. To enable the World Health Organization include appropriate G6PD POC diagnostic tests in its list of essential in-vitro diagnostics for use in resource-limited settings, we recommend a wider evaluation of available POC diagnostic tests for G6PD deficiency, particularly in malaria endemic countries.

Author Contributions: D.K. conceptualized the study and developed the analytical strategy. D.K. collected and processed the data, performed the statistical analysis, interpreted the results, and wrote the first draft of the study. D.A.A. assisted contributed to the data collection. K.M.A. contributed to the spatial analysis and interpretation of the results. T.P.M.-T., V.B., M.M., and P.K.D. contributed to the interpretation of the results, and did critical revisions. D.K. wrote the final draft. All authors have read and agree to the published version of the manuscript.

Funding: This research received no external funding.

Acknowledgments: We are thankful to the University of KwaZulu-Natal for providing us with essential research resources during this study. The authors would like to thank the authorities of the Upper East Regional Health Directorate, the District Health Management Teams, and all the rural PHC managers for granting us permission to conduct this study. We also thank the University of KwaZulu-Natal, College of Health Sciences for providing funding for the conduct of this study.

Conflicts of Interest: The authors declare no conflict of interest.

Abbreviations

ANC	Antenatal care
COVID-19	Coronavirus Disease 2019
G6PD	Glucose-6-Phosphate Dehydrogenase
GIS	Geographic Information Systems
PHC	Primary Healthcare
POC	Point-of-Care
RDT	Rapid Diagnostic Test
SDGs	Sustainable Development Goals
UER	Upper East Region
WHO	World Health Organization

References

1. Lee, J.; Kim, T.I.; Kang, J.-M.; Jun, H.; Lê, H.G.; Thái, T.L.; Sohn, W.-M.; Myint, M.K.; Lin, K.; Kim, T.-S.; et al. Prevalence of glucose-6-phosphate dehydrogenase (G6PD) deficiency among malaria patients in Upper Myanmar. *BMC Infect. Dis.* **2018**, *18*, 131. [CrossRef] [PubMed]
2. Beutler, E. Glucose-6-Phosphate Dehydrogenase Deficiency. *N. Engl. J. Med.* **1991**, *324*, 169–174. [PubMed]

3. Beutler, E. G6PD deficiency. *Blood* **1994**, *84*, 3613–3636. [CrossRef] [PubMed]
4. Nkhoma, E.T.; Poole, C.; Vannappagari, V.; Hall, S.A.; Beutler, E. The global prevalence of glucose-6-phosphate dehydrogenase deficiency: A systematic review and meta-analysis. *Blood Cells Mol. Dis.* **2009**, *42*, 267–278. [CrossRef]
5. Adu-Gyasi, D.; Asante, K.P.; Newton, S.; Dosoo, D.; Amoako, S.; Adjei, G.; Amoako, N.; Ankrah, L.; Tchum, S.K.; Mahama, E.; et al. Evaluation of the diagnostic accuracy of CareStart G6PD deficiency rapid diagnostic test (RDT) in a malaria endemic area in Ghana, Africa. *PLoS ONE* **2015**, *10*, e0125796. [CrossRef]
6. Hwang, S.; Mruk, K.; Rahighi, S.; Raub, A.G.; Chen, C.-H.; Dorn, L.E.; Horikoshi, N.; Wakatsuki, S.; Chen, J.; Mochly-Rosen, D. Correcting glucose-6-phosphate dehydrogenase deficiency with a small-molecule activator. *Nat. Commun.* **2018**, *9*, 4045. [CrossRef]
7. Luzzatto, L.; Seneca, E. G6PD deficiency: A classic example of pharmacogenetics with on-going clinical implications. *Br. J. Haematol.* **2013**, *164*, 469–480. [CrossRef]
8. Baird, J.K. Origins and implications of neglect of G6PD deficiency and primaquine toxicity inPlasmodium vivaxmalaria. *Pathog. Glob. Health* **2015**, *109*, 93–106. [CrossRef]
9. Vick, J.D. Chloroquine Is Not a Harmless Panacea for COVID-19—There's a Real Safety Concern with Malaria Drug USA: Medpagetoday. 2020. Available online: https://www.medpagetoday.com/infectiousdisease/covid19/85552 (accessed on 5 April 2020).
10. Gao, J.; Tian, Z.; Yang, X. Breakthrough: Chloroquine phosphate has shown apparent efficacy in treatment of COVID-19 associated pneumonia in clinical studies. *Biosci. Trends* **2020**, *14*, 72–73. [CrossRef]
11. Diallo, N.; Akweongo, P.; Maya, E.T.; Aikins, M.; Sarfo, B. Burden of malaria in mobile populations in the Greater Accra region, Ghana: A cross-sectional study. *Malar. J.* **2017**, *16*, 109. [CrossRef]
12. Owusu-Ofori, A.; Gadzo, D.; Bates, I. Transfusion-transmitted malaria: Donor prevalence of parasitaemia and a survey of healthcare workers knowledge and practices in a district hospital in Ghana. *Malar. J.* **2016**, *15*, 234. [CrossRef] [PubMed]
13. World Health Organisation. *Malaria Geneva: World Health Organisation*; WHO: Geneva, Switzerland, 2019. Available online: https://www.who.int/malaria/en/ (accessed on 4 August 2019).
14. World Health Organisation. *World Malaria Report 2018 Geneva: World Health Organisation*; WHO: Geneva, Switzerland, 2019. Available online: https://apps.who.int/iris/bitstream/handle/10665/275867/9789241565653-eng.pdf (accessed on 4 August 2019).
15. National Malaria Control Programme. *Intermittent Preventive Treatment in Pregnancy (IPTp) Accra: Ghana Health Service*. 2019. Available online: http://www.ghanahealthservice.org/malaria/item.php?nmcpiid=60&nmcpscid=114&nmcpcid=85 (accessed on 4 August 2019).
16. Van Eijk, A.M.; A Larsen, D.; Kayentao, K.; Koshy, G.; Slaughter, D.E.C.; Roper, C.; Okell, L.C.; Desai, M.; Gutman, J.; Khairallah, C.; et al. Effect of Plasmodium falciparum sulfadoxine-pyrimethamine resistance on the effectiveness of intermittent preventive therapy for malaria in pregnancy in Africa: A systematic review and meta-analysis. *Lancet Infect. Dis.* **2019**, *19*, 546–556. [CrossRef]
17. Kajubi, R.; Ochieng, T.; Kakuru, A.; Jagannathan, P.; Nakalembe, M.; Ruel, T.; Opira, B.; Ochokoru, H.; Ategeka, J.; Nayebare, P.; et al. Monthly sulfadoxine-pyrimethamine versus dihydroartemisinin-piperaquine for intermittent preventive treatment of malaria in pregnancy: A double-blind, randomised, controlled, superiority trial. *Lancet* **2019**, *393*, 1428–1439. [CrossRef]
18. Shulman, C.E.; Dorman, E.K.; Cutts, F.; Kawuondo, K.; Bulmer, J.N.; Peshu, N.; Marsh, K. Intermittent sulphadoxine-pyrimethamine to prevent severe anaemia secondary to malaria in pregnancy: A randomised placebo-controlled trial. *Lancet* **1999**, *353*, 632–636. [CrossRef]
19. Schultz, L.J.; Steketee, R.W.; Macheso, A.; Kazembe, P.; Chitsulo, L.; Wirima, J.J. The Efficacy of Antimalarial Regimens Containing Sulfadoxine-Pyrimethamine and/or Chloroquine in Preventing Peripheral and Placental Plasmodium falciparum Infection among Pregnant Women in Malawi. *Am. J. Trop. Med. Hyg.* **1994**, *51*, 515–522. [CrossRef]
20. Wilson, N.; Ceesay, F.K.; Obed, S.A.; Adjei, A.A.; Gyasi, R.K.; Rodney, P.; Ndjakani, Y.; Anderson, W.A.; Lucchi, N.W.; Stiles, J.K. Intermittent Preventive Treatment with Sulfadoxine-Pyrimethamine against Malaria and Anemia in Pregnant Women. *Am. J. Trop. Med. Hyg.* **2011**, *85*, 12–21. [CrossRef]
21. World Health Organisation. *Single Dose Primaquine as a Gametocytocide in Plasmodium Falciparum Malaria Geneva: World Health Organisation*; WHO: Geneva, Switzerland, 2012. Available online: https://www.who.int/malaria/pq_updated_policy_recommendation_en_102012.pdf (accessed on 8 August 2019).

22. Republic of Ghana. Anti-Malaria Drug Policy for Ghana Accra: Ministry of Health. 2009. Available online: https://www.ghanahealthservice.org/downloads/GHS_Antimalaria_drug_policy.pdf (accessed on 4 August 2019).
23. White, N.J.; Li, G.; Gao, Q.; Luzzatto, L. Rationale for recommending a lower dose of primaquine as a Plasmodium falciparum gametocytocide in populations where G6PD deficiency is common. *Malar. J.* **2012**, *11*, 418. [CrossRef]
24. Chan, T.K.; Todd, D.; Tso, S.C. Drug-induced haemolysis in glucose-6-phosphate dehydrogenase deficiency. *BMJ* **1976**, *2*, 1227–1229. [CrossRef]
25. Owusu, R.; Asante, K.P.; Mahama, E.; Awini, E.; Anyorigiya, T.; Dosoo, D.; Amu, A.; Jakpa, G.; Ofei, E.; Segbaya, S.; et al. Glucose-6-Phosphate Dehydrogenase Deficiency and Haemoglobin Drop after Sulphadoxine-Pyrimethamine Use for Intermittent Preventive Treatment of Malaria during Pregnancy in Ghana—A Cohort Study. *PLoS ONE* **2015**, *10*, 0136828. [CrossRef]
26. Carter, N.; Pamba, A.; Duparc, S.; Waitumbi, J. Frequency of glucose-6-phosphate dehydrogenase deficiency in malaria patients from six African countries enrolled in two randomized anti-malarial clinical trials. *Malar. J.* **2011**, *10*, 241. [CrossRef]
27. Owusu-Agyei, S.; Nettey, O.E.A.; Zandoh, C.; Sulemana, A.; Adda, R.; Amenga-Etego, S.; Mbacke, C. Demographic patterns and trends in Central Ghana: Baseline indicators from the Kintampo Health and Demographic Surveillance System. *Glob. Health Action* **2012**, *5*, 19033. [CrossRef] [PubMed]
28. Amoako, N.; Asante, K.P.; Adjei, G.; Awandare, G.A.; Bimi, L.; Owusu-Agyei, S. Associations between Red Cell Polymorphisms and Plasmodium falciparum Infection in the Middle Belt of Ghana. *PLoS ONE* **2014**, *9*, e112868. [CrossRef] [PubMed]
29. Kuupiel, D.; Tlou, B.; Bawontuo, V.; Mashamba-Thompson, T.P. Accessibility of pregnancy-related point-of-care diagnostic tests for maternal healthcare in rural primary healthcare facilities in Northern Ghana: A cross-sectional survey. *Heliyon* **2019**, *5*, e01236. [CrossRef] [PubMed]
30. Kuupiel, D.; Tlou, B.; Bawontuo, V.; Drain, P.K.; Mashamba-Thompson, T.P. Poor supply chain management and stock-outs of point-of-care diagnostic tests in Upper East Region's primary healthcare clinics, Ghana. *PLoS ONE* **2019**, *14*, e0211498. [CrossRef] [PubMed]
31. Kuupiel, D.; Bawontuo, V.; Donkoh, A.; Drain, P.K.; Mashamba-Thompson, T.P. Empirical Framework for Point-of-Care Diagnostics Supply Chain Management for Accessibility and Sustainability of Diagnostic Services in Ghana's Primary Health Care Clinics. *Point Care J. Near Patient Test. Technol.* **2019**, *18*, 72–75. [CrossRef]
32. Kuupiel, D.; Adu, K.M.; Bawontuo, V.; Mashamba-Thompson, T.P. Geographical Accessibility to District Hospitals/Medical Laboratories for Comprehensive Antenatal Point-of-Care Diagnostic Services in the Upper East Region, Ghana. *EClinicalMedicine* **2019**, *13*, 74–80. [CrossRef]
33. Ghana Statistical Service. *2010 Population & Housing Census: Summary Report of Final Results Accra: Ghana Statistical Service*; 2012. Available online: http://www.statsghana.gov.gh/docfiles/2010phc/Census2010_Summary_report_of_final_results.pdf (accessed on 25 January 2020).
34. Kuupiel, D.; Adu, K.; Apiribu, F.; Bawontuo, V.; Adogboba, D.; Ali, K.T.; Mashamba-Thompson, T.P. Geographic accessibility to public health facilities providing tuberculosis testing services at point-of-care in the upper east region, Ghana. *BMC Public Health* **2019**, *19*, 718. [CrossRef]
35. Becher, H.; Müller, O.; Jahn, A.; Gbangou, A.; Kynast-Wolf, G.; Kouyaté, B. Risk factors of infant and child mortality in rural Burkina Faso. *Bull. World Health Organ.* **2004**, *82*, 265–273.
36. Therrell, B.L.; Padilla, C.D.; Loeber, J.G.; Kneisser, I.; Saadallah, A.; Borrajo, G.J.; Adams, J. Current status of newborn screening worldwide: 2015. *Semin. Perinatol.* **2015**, *39*, 171–187. [CrossRef]
37. Anderle, A.; Bancone, G.; Domingo, G.J.; Gerth-Guyette, E.; Pal, S.; Satyagraha, A. Point-of-Care Testing for G6PD Deficiency: Opportunities for Screening. *Int. J. Neonatal Screen.* **2018**, *4*, 34. [CrossRef]
38. Ley, B.; Luter, N.; Espino, F.E.; Devine, A.; Kalnoky, M.; Lubell, Y.; Thriemer, K.; Baird, J.K.; Poirot, E.; Conan, N.; et al. The challenges of introducing routine G6PD testing into radical cure: A workshop report. *Malar. J.* **2015**, *14*, 377. [CrossRef] [PubMed]
39. Kuupiel, D.; Adu, K.; Bawontuo, V.; Adogboba, D.; Mashamba-Thompson, T.P. Estimating the Spatial Accessibility to Blood Group and Rhesus Type Point-of-Care Testing for Maternal Healthcare in Ghana. *Diagnostics* **2019**, *9*, 175. [CrossRef]

40. Kuliszkiewicz-Janus, M.; Zimny, A. Glucose-6-phosphate dehydrogenase (G6PD) deficiency—A cause of anaemia in pregnant women. *Pol. Arch. Intern. Med.* **2003**, *110*, 1327–1333.
41. WHO. *Coronavirus Disease (COVID-19) Pandemic Geneva: World Health Organization*. 2020. Available online: https://www.who.int/emergencies/diseases/novel-coronavirus-2019 (accessed on 5 April 2020).
42. Patel, A.; Waters, N. Using geographic information systems for health research. In *Application of Geographic Information Systems*; IntechOpen: London, UK, 2012.
43. Dangisso, M.H.; Datiko, D.G.; Lindtjørn, B. Accessibility to tuberculosis control services and tuberculosis programme performance in southern Ethiopia. *Glob. Health Action* **2015**, *8*, 29443. [CrossRef] [PubMed]
44. Kost, G.J. Theory, Principles, and Practice of Optimizing Point-of-Care Small-World Networks. *Point Care J. Near Patient Test. Technol.* **2012**, *11*, 96–101. [CrossRef]
45. Ferguson, W.J.; Kemp, K.; Kost, G.J. Using a geographic information system to enhance patient access to point-of-care diagnostics in a limited-resource setting. *Int. J. Health Geogr.* **2016**, *15*, 10. [CrossRef]
46. Kost, G.J. Geospatial Science and Point-of-Care Testing: Creating Solutions for Population Access, Emergencies, Outbreaks, and Disasters. *Front. Public Health* **2019**, *7*, 329. [CrossRef]
47. Arthur, E. Wealth and antenatal care use: Implications for maternal health care utilisation in Ghana. *Health Econ. Rev.* **2012**, *2*, 14. [CrossRef]
48. Gething, P.W.; Johnson, F.A.; Frempong-Ainguah, F.; Nyarko, P.; Baschieri, A.; Aboagye, P.; Falkingham, J.; Matthews, Z.; Atkinson, P.M. Geographical access to care at birth in Ghana: A barrier to safe motherhood. *BMC Public Health* **2012**, *12*, 991. [CrossRef]

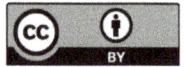

© 2020 by the authors. Licensee MDPI, Basel, Switzerland. This article is an open access article distributed under the terms and conditions of the Creative Commons Attribution (CC BY) license (http://creativecommons.org/licenses/by/4.0/).

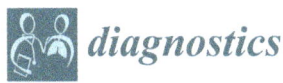

Article

Estimating the Spatial Accessibility to Blood Group and Rhesus Type Point-of-Care Testing for Maternal Healthcare in Ghana

Desmond Kuupiel [1,2,*], Kwame M. Adu [3], Vitalis Bawontuo [2,4], Duncan A. Adogboba [5] and Tivani P. Mashamba-Thompson [1]

1. Discipline of Public Health Medicine, School 0.0of Nursing and Public Health, University of KwaZulu-Natal, Durban 4001, South Africa; Mashamba-Thompson@ukzn.ac.za
2. Research for Sustainable Development Consult, Sunyani, Ghana; bawontuovitalis@yahoo.com
3. Adu Manu Kwame Consult, Accra, Ghana; meous007@gmail.com
4. Faculty of Health and Allied Sciences, Catholic University College of Ghana, Fiapre, Sunyani, Ghana
5. Regional Health Directorate, Ghana Health Service, Upper East Region, Bolgatanga, Ghana; alemna@gmail.com
* Correspondence: desmondkuupiel98@hotmail.com or KuupielD@ukzn.ac.za; Tel.: +27-735568200 or +233-550972968

Received: 29 September 2019; Accepted: 29 October 2019; Published: 5 November 2019

Abstract: Background: In Ghana, a blood group and rhesus type test is one of the essential recommended screening tests for women during antenatal care since blood transfusion is a key intervention for haemorrhage. We estimated the spatial accessibility to health facilities for blood group and type point-of-care (POC) testing in the Upper East Region (UER), Ghana. Methods: We assembled the attributes and spatial data of hospitals, clinics, and medical laboratories providing blood group and rhesus type POC testing in the UER. We also obtained the spatial data of all the 131 towns, and 94 health centres and community-based health planning and services (CHPS) compounds providing maternal healthcare in the region. We further obtained the topographical data of the region, and travel time estimated using an assumed tricycle speed of 20 km/h. We employed ArcGIS 10.5 to estimate the distance and travel time and locations with poor spatial access identified for priority improvement. Findings: In all, blood group and rhesus type POC testing was available in 18 health facilities comprising eight public hospitals and six health centres, one private hospital, and three medical laboratories used as referral points by neighbouring health centres and CHPS compounds without the service. Of the 94 health centres and CHPS compounds, 51.1% (48/94) and 66.4% (87/131) of the towns were within a 10 km range to a facility providing blood group and rhesus type testing service. The estimated mean distance to a health facility for blood group and rhesus POC testing was 8.9 ± 4.1 km, whilst the mean travel time was 17.8 ± 8.3 min. Builsa South district recorded the longest mean distance (25.6 ± 7.4 km), whilst Bongo district recorded the shortest (3.1 ± 1.9 km). The spatial autocorrelation results showed the health facilities providing blood group and rhesus type POC testing were randomly distributed in the region (Moran Index = 0.29; z-score = 1.37; $p = 0.17$). Conclusion: This study enabled the identification of district variations in spatial accessibility to blood group and rhesus type POC testing in the region for policy decisions. We urge the health authorities in Ghana to evaluate and implement recommended POC tests such as slide agglutination tests for blood group and rhesus type testing in resource-limited settings.

Keywords: spatial accessibility; blood group; rhesus type; point-of-care testing; maternal healthcare; Upper East Region; Ghana

1. Introduction

Since 1990, the world has made significant progress in reducing maternal mortality [1]. Despite the progress made, recent evidence shows that every eleven seconds a pregnant woman dies somewhere in the world according to the World Health Organisation (WHO) [1]. In 2017, approximately 295,000 women died from mostly preventable causes during and subsequent to pregnancy and childbirth; 94% of these mortalities occurred in resource-limited settings [2]. Sub-Saharan Africa (SSA) and Southern Asia alone accounted for 86% of all maternal deaths in the world [2]. The WHO estimates show that in 2017, SSA countries including Ghana alone accounted for almost two-thirds (196,000) of maternal deaths compared to Southern Asia which accounted for approximately one-fifth (58,000) [2]. Haemorrhage remains a major direct cause of maternal death and together with hypertensive disorders and sepsis accounts for more than 50% maternal deaths globally [3]. A recent global systematic review by Say and colleagues revealed that haemorrhage accounted for about 27.1% ahead of hypertensive disorders with 14%, and sepsis (10.7%) of the total 60,799 maternal deaths retrieved from 23 eligible studies published from 2003 to 2012 [3]. Blood transfusion service is one of the critical interventions for the management of haemorrhage [4].

Blood transfusion saves lives and improves health, but many patients, including pregnant women or women during delivery, requiring transfusion do not have timely access to safe blood [5]. A blood transfusion may become crucial at any time in both urban and rural communities [5]. Improving access to safe blood transfusion relies partly on the ability of the health facility to effectively perform point-of-care (POC) testing for blood group and rhesus type. Generally, access to healthcare services including blood group and rhesus type POC testing may also be influenced by several factors such as the availability of laboratory services, human resource capacity, availability of POC tests and supply chain management of the diagnostic tests, cost, wealth, quality of care, occupation, cultural practices, education, and the location of the service [6–9]. The nature of the road and networks, type of transport systems, topology, land use, building use, traffic condition and population density, and seasonal variations may also influence travel time to healthcare facilities, particularly in rural areas [7,10]. In some settings, these factors may interact in a complex way and geographical access in terms of distance and travel time may be insignificant [7]. Nonetheless, where the availability of POC testing for blood group and rhesus type is poor and laboratory services are sparse, the geographical location of the service becomes a key barrier to the service, particularly for the rural populations and, hence, very essential [7,11–13].

In Ghana, evidence shows that the maternal mortality ratio presently stands at 319 per 100,000 live births [1,13–15]. Haemorrhage is one of the direct causes of maternal deaths in Ghana and among the top five causes [16,17]. The Der et al. study in 2013 identified haemorrhage as the topmost cause of maternal mortality in Ghana accounting for 21.8% of all deaths with abortion, hypertensive disorders, infections, and ectopic gestation accounting for 20.7%, 19.4%, 9.1%, and 8.7%, respectively [17]. Many interventions including the implementation of a free maternal healthcare policy since 2003, provision of emergency obstetric care, expansions of health infrastructure, increased training of midwives and posting them to underserved communities, and ongoing investment in primary healthcare (PHC) facilities such as health centres and community-based health planning and service (CHPS) facilities are meant to reduce maternal deaths in the country. Pregnant women in Ghana are also expected to undertake a blood type screening test as part of the wide range of healthcare services rendered to them during the first antenatal care (ANC) visit irrespective of the level of care [18,19]. Like most SSA countries, Ghana's PHC facilities often do not have laboratories to perform blood type screening tests for patients and donors as well as facilities for safe storage of blood. In 2018, a cross-sectional study was conducted aimed to investigate the availability and use of pregnancy-related point-of-care (POC) tests in Ghana's PHC clinics [20]. Of the 100 participating PHC clinics in the survey, blood group and rhesus type testing was available in only six clinics with some form of laboratory services in the Upper East Region (UER) [20]. Whilst the average ANC clinic attendance per month was shown to be 65 pregnant women with a minimum of 30 and a maximum of 360 [20]. The results of the survey also revealed that out of the 94 clinics without blood group and rhesus type testing, 89 demonstrated the need for it in their clinics [20]. The findings of the survey revealed blood group and rhesus type testing is still a laboratory-based test in Ghana performed by trained laboratory professionals and, hence, may not be accessible to all who need it [20].

Despite this, to date, no study has measured the spatial accessibility in terms of distance and travel time to health facilities providing blood type testing services in Ghana, especially in the UER. Knowledge of the distance and travel time to the nearest health facility for a blood type screening test is potentially essential to help the Government of Ghana implement POC testing services in rural health facilities located in geographical settings with poor access as recommended by the WHO and bring healthcare closer to where people live and work [21]. We, therefore, investigated the spatial accessibility to blood group and rhesus type POC testing during ANC in the UER of Ghana.

2. Methods

2.1. Overview

This is a follow-up on our previously published cross-sectional study which investigated the availability and use of pregnancy-related POC tests in the UER utilising a hundred PHC clinics (health centres and CHPS compounds) randomly selected from a total of 356 clinics from all the districts in the region [20]. The sampling strategy used to select the 100 PHC clinics as well as the study area (UER) has been adequately described in the previously published survey [20]. The survey revealed that of the 100 PHC clinics, blood type screening test was available only in six clinics, and all six were health centres with some form of laboratory services [20]. To measure the spatial accessibility to health facilities where blood type screening testing is available in the regions, the cost-distance algorithm was applied using the ArcGIS desktop software. The flow diagram (Figure 1) illustrates the data, methods, and models used. All the attributes and spatial data used for this study were obtained in 2018.

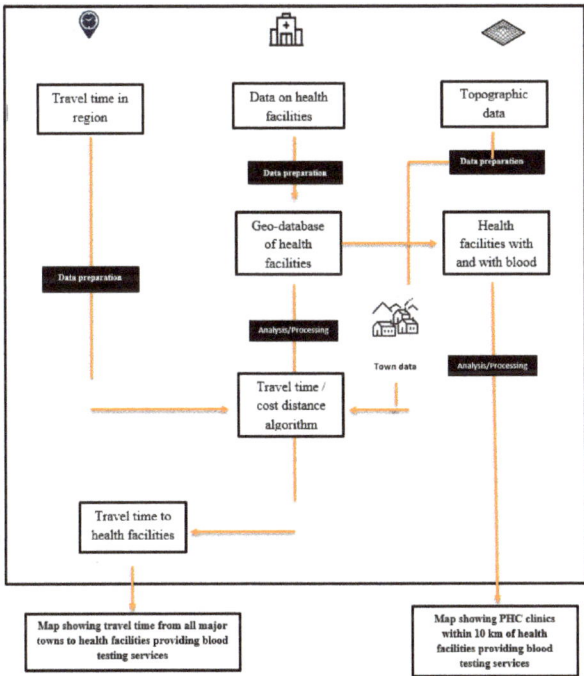

Figure 1. A flow diagram illustrating the data, methods, and models used. PHC—primary healthcare.

We extracted the attribute data on all the 100 PHC clinics and health facilities where expectant mothers (who require blood group and rhesus status testing) were referred for blood type screening tests during ANC. These data which were obtained in text data format were loaded into the ArcGIS 10.5 software and transformed into a shapefile to allow for performing spatial analysis using ArcGIS. The topographic data gathered for this current study included roads, rivers, and the slope obtained as the digital elevation model (DEM). The topographical data were obtained for the whole of West Africa and the UER processed as a subset of Ghana. Road data were obtained to inform travel routes and, in view of this, types of roads were appended as attribute data to the spatial data to inform the potential speed users are likely to experience on each road type which may as well greatly inform travel distance and time. The DEM for the West Africa region was obtained to inform the slope of every location in the UER. This was necessary because identifying valleys and hills was key to determining which areas serve as barriers and are inaccessible to users. The DEM dataset was obtained from Adu Manu Kwame (AMK) Consultancy and compared with the data obtained from the University of Ghana Remote Sensing and Geographic Information Systems Laboratory for accuracy. We then reclassified the slope data into highlands (more than 200 m high) and flatlands (between 119 and 200 m high) as informed by the DEM data which showed that the highest point in the UER was about 470 m, and 119 m was the lowest point.

2.2. Spatial Data of Health Facilities

To realise the objectives of this study, the geo-location data of all the 100 PHC clinics and health facilities such as public hospitals or clinics offering blood type testing services as well as private medical laboratories or hospital/clinics being utilised as referral points for blood type testing services were obtained from the Regional Health Directorate of the Ghana Health Service, UER. We also obtained the spatial data of all the 131 towns in the region using the global positioning system. To accurately map all the latitude and longitude to their relative location on the earth, the World Geodetic System 30 North coordinate system was applied to the entire dataset because Ghana falls within this zone.

2.3. Geospatial Analysis

Developing a Model for Estimating the Travel Time

As a key aspect of this study, the model for determining the travel time was carefully developed taking into consideration all the datasets. Using the PyScripter integrated development environment and relying on the Python capabilities of ArcGIS 5.0, a model was developed to calculate the travel time and for data transformation. The cost distance model which calculates the shortest time to a source based on a cost dataset was used to determine distance. A motorised tricycle was identified as the commonly used public transport for travel within UER, hence, travel time was estimated via road and via paths and tracks using an assumed motorised tricycle speed of 20 km per hour. We recalibrated travel time per pixel (10 m × 10 m grid) for both roads and paths to enable estimation of travel time from PHC clinics where blood type testing services are not available to the nearest hospital, clinic, or medical laboratory for all the districts in the region. Although travel time can be influenced by many factors, we chose to estimate travel time via roads and paths because they are the commonly used routes in the region. Likewise, the motorised transport system was chosen because we found it was the most used public mode of transport for journeys within the region. The model and procedure used to approximate the travel time for this current study have been published in our previous studies focusing on geographical access to tuberculosis diagnostic services and comprehensive ANC POC diagnostic services [12,13]. Supplementary file 1 presents a detailed description of the procedure.

2.4. Buffer

We employed the geospatial analysis proximity tool (Buffer) to identify towns and PHC clinics without a blood group and rhesus type testing service located within a 10 km radius, and those located beyond 10 km to a health facility providing the service. We additionally estimated the proximity of all the 131 towns to the nearest health facility providing blood group and rhesus type testing service. Evidence shows that access to healthcare elsewhere more than 10 km away is associated with higher risks of poor health outcomes [22]. 'Buffer' in geographic information systems (GIS) refers to a boundary defined by specific units that surround a source or feature. For the purposes of this study, the point buffer was employed because the origin feature in this study which is health facilities providing blood type testing service is a point feature (vector dataset).

To assess the accuracy, we created a set of random points from the ground truth data and compared that to the classified data in a confusion matrix using three geoprocessing tools: create accuracy assessment points, update accuracy assessment points, and compute confusion matrix.

2.5. Spatial Autocorrelation

We utilised the spatial autocorrelation tool in ArcMap 10.5 to determine the spatial distribution of the health facilities providing blood type testing services in the region. Spatial autocorrelation mirrors the first law of geography which states that "everything is related to everything else, but near things are more related than distant things" [23]. In spatial autocorrelation, the null hypothesis of the Moran's Index statistic states that the feature being measured is distributed randomly, however, when the p-value obtained from running the spatial analyst tool proves to be statistically significant, then the null hypothesis can be rejected [24]. Guided by this, we considered a positive correlation to mean similar values clustered together while negative correlation is representative of different values clustered in a location, and zero means no correlation.

2.6. Ethics Approval

This study was approved by the Navrongo Health Research Centre Institutional Review Board/Ghana Health Service (approval number: NHRCIRB291) on 8th January 2018 and the University of KwaZulu-Natal Biomedical Research Ethics Committee (approval number: BE565/17) on 12th February 2018

3. Results

3.1. Characteristics of the Health Facilities Providing Blood Group and Rhesus Type POC Testing

In all, blood group and rhesus type POC testing was available in 18 health facilities. Of the 18 health facilities, nine (50%) were hospitals and six (33.3%) health centres. The remaining three (16.7%) health facilities were private medical laboratories which were used as referral points by some of the PHC clinics without blood group and rhesus type POC testing service. Of the nine hospitals providing blood group and rhesus type POC testing services, the majority (77.8%) are owned and managed by the Ghana Health Service (GHS), 11.1% are owned and managed by the Christian Health Association of Ghana (CHAG), and 11.1% by private individuals. Similarly, 83.3% (5/6) of the sub-district health centres offering blood group and rhesus type POC testing are owned and managed by GHS, whilst one (16.7%) is owned by CHAG. All the 18 health facilities offering blood group and rhesus type POC testing services were distributed across nine out of the 13 districts in the region. Four (22.2%) each were in the Bongo district and Bolgatanga municipality; meanwhile, there was no health facility providing blood group and rhesus type POC testing services in Builsa South, Nabdam, Binduri, and Pusiga districts (Figure 2).

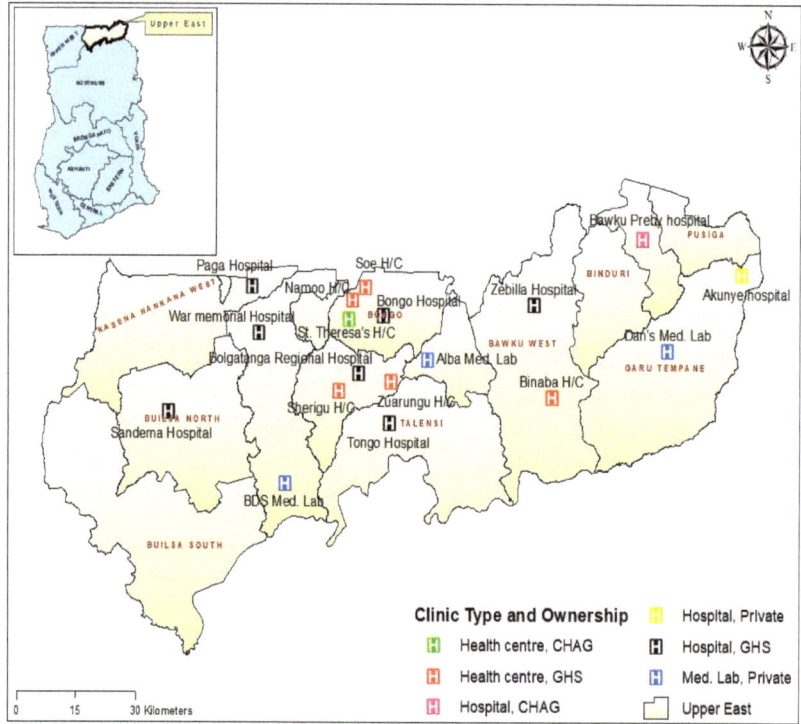

Figure 2. Map showing the geographical location, facility type, and ownership of health facilities providing blood type testing services in the Upper East Region (UER). CHAG—Christian Health Association of Ghana; GHS—Ghana Health Services.

3.2. Spatial Distribution of Health Facilities Providing Blood Grouping and Rhesus Type Testing Services in the UER

To determine the spatial distribution of health facilities providing blood grouping and rhesus type testing services in the region, spatial autocorrelation analysis was conducted. The results showed a positive spatial autocorrelation (Moran Index = 0.29; z-score = 1.37; p = 0.17) suggesting that health facilities providing blood group and rhesus type testing services were randomly distributed spatially in the region (Figure 3).

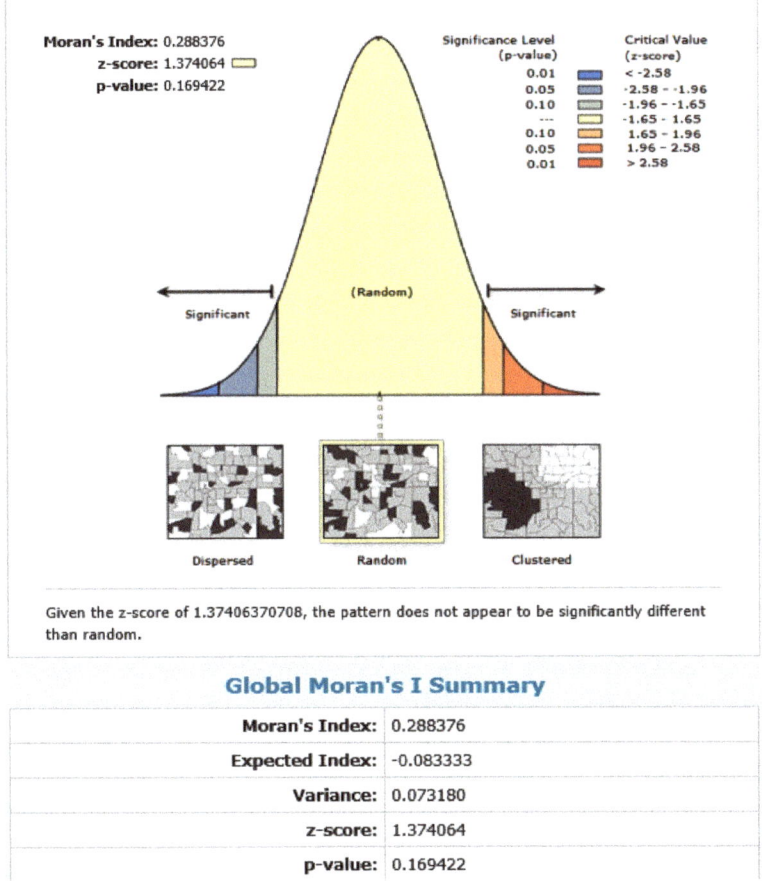

Figure 3. Spatial autocorrelation map showing the spatial distribution of health facilities providing blood group and rhesus type testing in the UER.

3.3. Spatial Accessibility to Blood Group and Rhesus Type Testing in the UER

We estimated the proximity (distance) of the 94 PHC clinics without blood group and rhesus type testing service from the previous cross-sectional study to the nearest health facility providing blood group and rhesus type testing services in the region. The results showed that 48 (51.1%) of the PHC clinics without blood group and rhesus type testing service were within 10 km reach to the nearest health facility offering the services. All the participating PHC clinics without blood group and rhesus type testing service from Bolgatanga Municipal and Bongo district were within 10 km range to the closest facility providing the service. However, none of the PHC clinics included in this study from the Builsa South district were within 10 km reach of any of the health facilities providing blood group and rhesus type testing service (Figure 4).

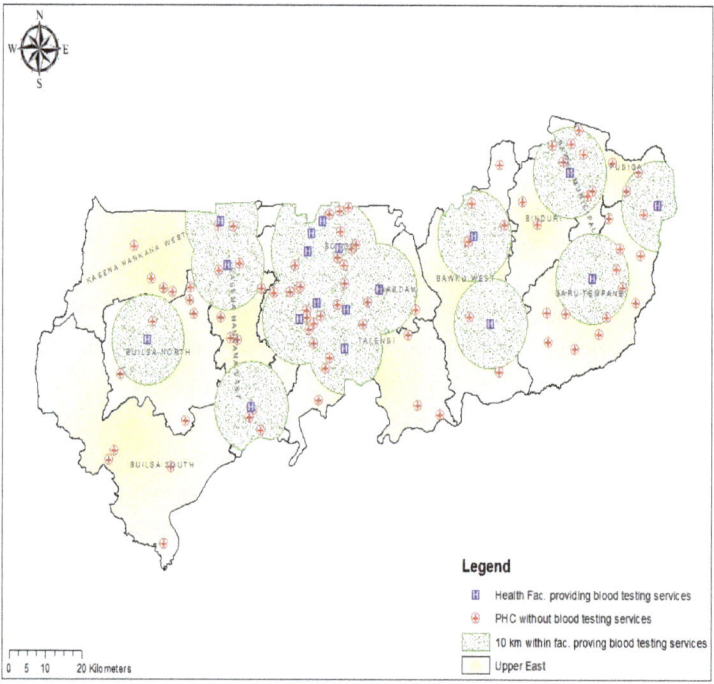

Figure 4. Map showing the distribution of the PHC clinics and distance within 10 km from the nearest health facility providing blood group and rhesus type testing services in the UER.

Based on the PHC clinics included in this analysis, the mean (standard deviation (SD)) distance from a PHC clinic without blood group and rhesus type testing service to the closest facility providing the service in the UER was 12.6 ± 5.2 km. The longest mean distance was recorded in the Builsa South (32.2 ± 13.2 km) district, whilst the shortest (3.3 ± 1.4 km) was in the Bongo district. The results also show that the mean travel time from a PHC clinic without blood group and rhesus type testing service to the closest facility providing the service in the UER was 37.7 ± 15.4 min. Again, Builsa South district recorded the longest travel time (96 ± 39.4 min), whilst Bongo district recorded the shortest travel time (9.9 ± 4.1 min) to the nearest facility offering blood group and rhesus type testing service (Figure 5).

This study also estimated the proximity of all the 131 towns to their nearest health facilities providing blood group and rhesus type testing services. The results showed that 87 (66.4%) of the towns were within a 10 km radius (less than 30 min travel time) to a health facility providing blood group and rhesus type testing service. Twenty-five (19.1%) of the 131 towns were located between 10 and 15 km to a health facility offering blood group and rhesus type testing service, whilst 15 (11.5%) towns were located at more than 15–25 km reach. Meanwhile, 4 (3.1%) towns in Builsa South district were found to be located more than 25 km to the nearest health facility providing blood group and rhesus type testing service (Figure 6). Supplementary file 2 provides the distance/travel time categorisation of the towns and their names.

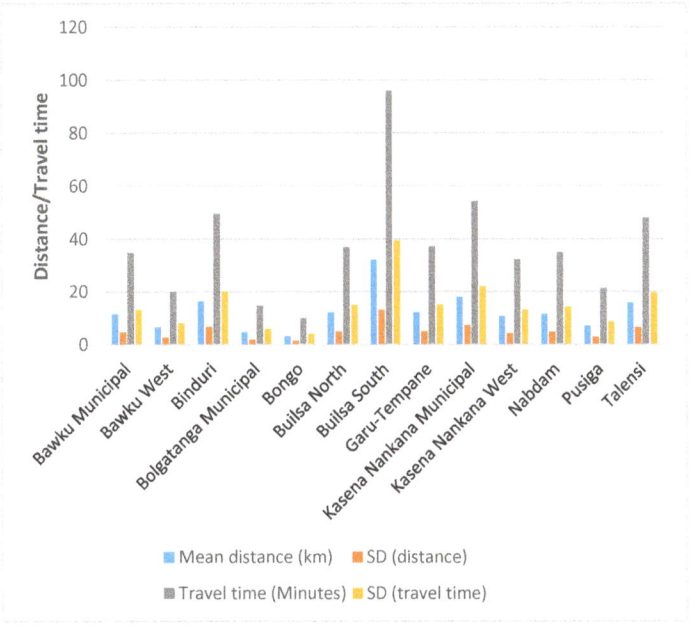

Figure 5. A bar chart depicting the mean distance and travel time from PHC clinics to the nearest health facility providing blood group and rhesus type testing services per district in the UER.

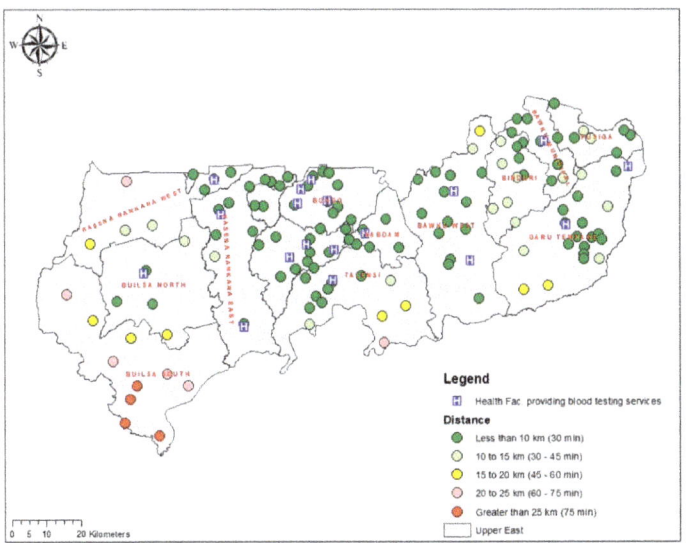

Figure 6. Map showing the distribution of distance (km) and travel time (minutes) from towns to health facilities providing blood group and rhesus type testing services in the UER.

This study's findings further showed that the mean distance and travel time ± SD from all locations in the 131 towns of the UER to a health facility providing blood group and rhesus type testing service in the region was 8.9 ± 4.1 km and the mean travel time was 17.8 ± 8.3 min. Builsa South and Bongo districts once again recorded the longest mean distance (25.6 ± 7.4 km) and the shortest

(3.1 ± 1.9 km), respectively, to a health facility providing blood group and rhesus testing service in the region. Similarly, the mean travel time from all locations in the 131 towns of the UER to a health facility providing blood group and rhesus type testing services in the region was estimated at 17.8 ± 8.3 min with Builsa South district recording the longest travel time (51.3 ± 14.8 min) and the shortest time recorded in Bongo district (6.2 ± 3.9 min) (Figure 7).

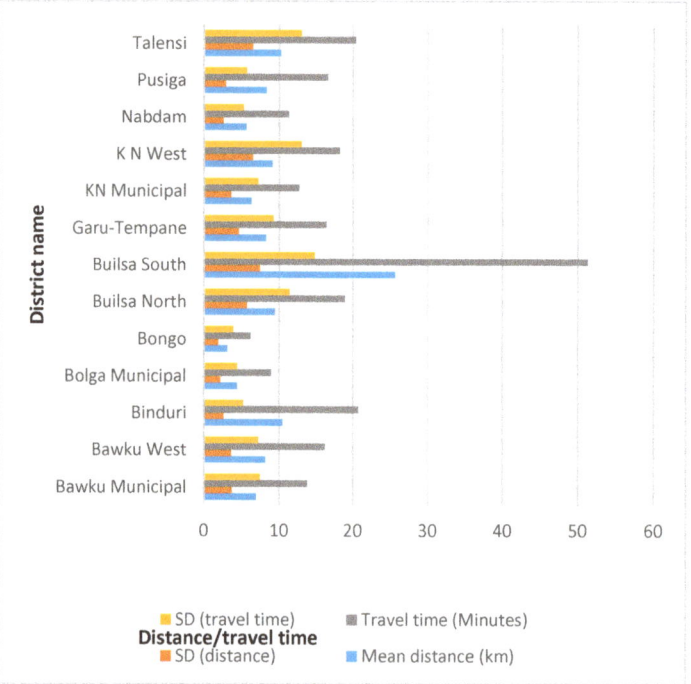

Figure 7. A bar chart depicting the mean distance and travel time from all 131 towns in the UER to a health facility providing blood group and rhesus type testing services per district in the region.

4. Discussion

This study estimated the spatial accessibility (distance and travel time) to health facilities for blood group and rhesus type testing during ANC in the UER of Ghana. The results showed the about 51.1% of the PHC clinics without blood group and rhesus type testing and 66.4% of the towns in the region were within 10 km range to a facility providing the service. The mean distance to a health facility providing blood group and rhesus type testing service in the region was 8.9 ± 4.1 km, whilst the mean travel time was 17.8 ± 8.3 min using a motorised tricycle speed of 20 km/hour. The results further showed that the spatial autocorrelation of the health facilities providing blood group and rhesus type testing services were randomly distributed in the region.

We found the majority of the PHC clinics without blood group and rhesus type testing and the towns in the UER were within 10 km proximity to the nearest health facility providing the service. Although this finding is fairly good, at the same time, it depicts that almost half (48.9%) of the PHC clinics are without blood group and rhesus type testing facilities; moreover, about 33.6% of the towns are still geo-located beyond 10 km to a facility providing the services. This could also result in low utilisation of blood group and rhesus type testing services, overcrowding at the health facilities, and increased waiting time for test results. Evidence shows that people tend to limit the use of health services to facilities closer to them [25]. Ferguson and colleagues also demonstrated that having diagnostic technologies closer to populations streamlines critical care paths [26]. Hence, these results have revealed the need to equip the PHC clinics to enable them to provide POC testing for blood group and rhesus type tests in the region. Contrary to this current study finding, a previous study in the UER reported fewer PHC clinics were within 10 km reach to either a hospital or medical laboratory for a one-stop ANC POC diagnostic service [13].

We also found the mean distance to blood group and rhesus type POC testing in the region to be 8.9 ± 4.1 km and a mean travel time of 17.8 ± 8.3 min using a motorised tricycle speed of 20 km/hour. These findings suggest moderate spatial accessibility to blood group and rhesus type testing. It is possible that a substantial proportion of women of reproductive age live beyond 8.9 km from nearest health facility providing the service. The distance of 8.9 km and can take several hours for a pregnant woman to walk in the case where she is unable to afford the services of a motorised tricycle. Even when a pregnant woman can afford the services of a motorised tricycle but considering the bad state of the roads in the region, particularly in the rural areas, the speed of the tricycle may be less than the average 20 km/h used in our analysis. Therefore, the travel time to the nearest health facility may exceed the estimated travel time we found in some cases. In this case, it is possible that a significant number of referred pregnant women from PHC clinics may not go to the referral facilities for blood group and rhesus type testing during ANC and this potentially could become problematic when the need arises for urgent blood transfusion. Although we found no other study demonstrating evidence on spatial accessibility to health facilities for blood group and rhesus type testing, Gething and colleagues' study on geographical access to care at birth in Ghana reported longer journey times to emergency obstetric and neonatal care [7]. Likewise, a study in South Africa by Tanser and colleagues also demonstrated poor physical accessibility (travel time of 170 min) to healthcare [10].

We further found the spatial autocorrelation findings also demonstrated the health facilities providing blood group and rhesus type testing services were randomly distributed in the region. This suggests the health facilities were neither clustered nor dispersed in the UER. However, our analysis showed district-wise variation in spatial accessibility to public hospitals and clinics offering blood group and rhesus type POC testing services in the region. Nonetheless, we have highlighted worst-served areas for improvement by the health authorities to address the disparities revealed, particularly, in the Builsa South district. Similarly, our previous studies in the UER which assessed the geographical access to a comprehensive ANC and tuberculosis POC testing also found geographic variations of the health facilities with moderate accessibility to diagnostic services [12,13].

Knowledge of blood group and rhesus type is of paramount importance to prevent transfusion-related complications particularly among pregnant mothers [27]. However, the findings revealed a low number of PHC facilities providing ABO and rhesus factor testing resulting in spatial variation of the service provision. Possible solutions to the geographical access and/or knowledge gap of pregnant mothers on ABO and rhesus factor type may include the implementation of POC testing for blood group and rhesus type in Ghana's PHC clinics in accordance with the WHO recommendation. The WHO recommends a slide agglutination test using capillary whole blood or venous whole blood to determine A, B, and O groups and Rh type in resource-limited settings to facilitate the screening of patients, donors, safe blood transfusion, and improve access to healthcare and outcomes [21]. This will enable every pregnant woman and blood donors to be screened during ANC services for safe blood transfusion when needed urgently. The implementation of POC testing for blood group and rhesus type in Ghana's PHC clinics may well reduce the distance and travel time to help improve access to healthcare generally and better maternal health outcomes in resource-limited settings. Additionally, the cost and risks of traveling long distances to access blood group and rhesus type testing services potentially will be reduced with a resultant increase in utilisation. Moreover, the implementation of POC testing of blood grouping and rhesus type for maternal healthcare may lead to a reduction of maternal deaths caused by haemorrhage, hence contributing to Ghana's achievement of Sustainable Development Goal 3.1 (less than 70 maternal deaths per 100,000 live births) by 2030. According to WHO, countries such as Belarus, Bangladesh, Cambodia, Kazakhstan, Malawi, Morocco, Mongolia,

Rwanda, Timor-Leste, and Zambia made substantial progress in reducing maternal mortality owing to the implementation of several interventions including their focus on improving the quality of care at the PHC level and universal health coverage [1].

Using geographical information systems (GIS) to inform the implementation of health services has been shown to be useful [28–30]. GIS effectively enables implementation of POC testing in health networks to streamline decision making at the POC [26]. Hence, GIS helps improve patient health outcomes, save time and money, and ensure that the health networks are sufficiently resourced to deliver needed health services to the population [26]. Despite these strengths, there are several limitations worth noting such as our inability to include non-spatial factors in the analysis. Non-spatial factors such as the income of patients [8], age, cultural practices, education, and others can also influence the utilisation of health services even if the service is very close to the individual [7]. Although the implementation of POC testing for blood group and rhesus type testing in PHC clinics has the potential to improve maternal health outcomes, this study did not assess the cost–benefit analysis and other challenges associated with the implementation. Nonetheless, knowledge of one's blood group and rhesus type and safe blood transfusion timely could save many lives including those of pregnant women before, during, and after delivery. The travel time estimation provided by this study was dependent on only one mode of transportation using an assumed speed which might be inaccurate. Moreover, this study was limited to only one region in Ghana, and, therefore, the findings may not necessarily apply to the remaining fifteen regions in the country. We therefore recommend future research to focus on areas such as the non-spatial factors and cost–benefit analysis of implementing POC testing for blood group and rhesus type in PHC clinics. We also recommend a similar study in the other fifteen regions of Ghana. Notwithstanding these limitations, this study has provided evidence-based information useful for policy decision-making for targeted improvement of POC testing for blood group and rhesus type testing in the UER. Since this study is the first, it may possibly stimulate more research using GIS to evaluate access to blood group and rhesus type testing services in other similar settings for improving healthcare.

5. Conclusions

A blood group and rhesus type test are a prerequisite for both blood recipients and donors prior to transfusion to prevent or reduce blood-transfusion-related complications. The current mean distance and travel time to health facilities for blood group and rhesus type testing service in the UER is estimated at 8.9 ± 4.1 km, whilst the mean travel time was 17.8 ± 8.3 min using a motorised tricycle speed of 20 km/hour. This distance and travel time possibly may reduce substantially if blood group and rhesus type POC testing services are implemented in PHC clinics, particularly in those districts with poor spatial access evidenced by this study. We recommend the establishment and implementation of an essential diagnostic list including POC tests for blood group and rhesus type test in Ghana in line with the WHO recommendation to help address diagnostic challenges in resource-limited settings.

Supplementary Materials: The following are available online at http://www.mdpi.com/2075-4418/9/4/175/s1, Supplementary file 1: Procedure for estimating the travel time, Supplementary file 2: Distance/travel time categorisation of the towns and their names.

Author Contributions: D.K. conceptualised the study and developed the analytical strategy. D.K. collected and processed the data, performed statistical analysis, interpreted the results, and wrote the first draft of the study. K.M.A. contributed to the spatial analysis and interpretation of the results. T.P.M.-T. and V.B. contributed to the analytical strategy, to the interpretation of the results, and did critical revisions. D.K. wrote the final draft and it was approved by all authors.

Acknowledgments: We are thankful to the University of KwaZulu-Natal for providing us with essential research resources during this study. The authors would like to thank the authorities of the Upper East Regional Health Directorate, the District Health Management Teams, and all the rural PHC managers for granting us permission to conduct this study. We also thank the University of KwaZulu-Natal, College of Health Sciences for providing funding for the conduct of this study.

Conflicts of Interest: The authors declare no conflict of interest.

Abbreviations

ANC	Antenatal care
CHAG	Christian Health Association of Ghana
DEM	Digital elevation model
GHS	Ghana Health Service
GIS	Geographic Information Systems
PHC	Primary healthcare
POC	Point-of-care
SSA	Sub-Saharan Africa
UER	Upper East Region
WHO	World Health Organisation

References

1. World Health Organisation. More Women and Children Survive Today than ever before—UN Report. Available online: https://www.who.int/news-room/detail/19-09-2019-more-women-and-children-survive-today-than-ever-before-un-report (accessed on 20 September 2019).
2. World Health Organization. Trends in Maternal Mortality: 2000 to 2017: Estimates by WHO, UNICEF, UNFPA, World Bank Group and the United Nations Population Division. Available online: http://documents.worldbank.org/curated/en/793971568908763231/pdf/Trends-in-maternal-mortality-2000-to-2017-Estimates-by-WHO-UNICEF-UNFPA-World-Bank-Group-and-the-United-Nations-Population-Division.pdf (accessed on 21 September 2019).
3. Say, L.; Chou, D.; Gemmill, A.; Tuncalp, O.; Moller, A.B.; Daniels, J.; Gulmezoglu, A.M.; Temmerman, M.; Alkema, L. Global causes of maternal death: a WHO systematic analysis. *Lancet Glob. Health* **2014**, *2*, e323–e333. [CrossRef]
4. Ramani, K.V.; Mavalankar, D.V.; Govil, D. Study of blood-transfusion services in Maharashtra and Gujarat States, India. *J. Health Popul. Nutr.* **2009**, *27*, 259–270. [CrossRef] [PubMed]
5. World Health Organization. Blood Transfusion Safety. Available online: https://www.who.int/bloodsafety/testing_processing/components/en/ (accessed on 16 October 2019).
6. Guagliardo, M.F. Spatial accessibility of primary care: concepts, methods and challenges. *Int. J. Health Geogr* **2004**, *3*, 3. [CrossRef] [PubMed]
7. Gething, P.W.; Johnson, F.A.; Frempong-Ainguah, F.; Nyarko, P.; Baschieri, A.; Aboagye, P.; Falkingham, J.; Matthews, Z.; Atkinson, P.M. Geographical access to care at birth in Ghana: a barrier to safe motherhood. *BMC Public Health* **2012**, *12*, 991. [CrossRef] [PubMed]
8. Arthur, E. Wealth and antenatal care use: implications for maternal health care utilisation in Ghana. *Health Econ. Rev.* **2012**, *2*, 14. [CrossRef] [PubMed]
9. Kuupiel, D.; Bawontuo, V.; Mashamba-Thompson, T.P. Improving the Accessibility and Efficiency of Point-of-Care Diagnostics Services in Low- and Middle-Income Countries: Lean and Agile Supply Chain Management. *Diagnostics* **2017**, *7*, 58. [CrossRef] [PubMed]
10. Tanser, F.; Gijsbertsen, B.; Herbst, K. Modelling and understanding primary health care accessibility and utilization in rural South Africa: An exploration using a geographical information system. *Soc. Sci. Med. (1982)* **2006**, *63*, 691–705. [CrossRef] [PubMed]
11. MacKinney, A.; Coburn, A.; Lundblad, J.; McBride, T.; Mueller, K.; Watson, S. Access to Rural Health Care–A Literature Review and New Synthesis. *Policy Report. Rupri: Rural Policy Res. Inst.* **2014**. Available online: https://www.rupri.org/?library=access-to-rural-health-care-a-literature-review-and-new-synthesis-report-prepared-by-the-rupri-health-panel-august-2014 (accessed on 16 October 2019).
12. Kuupiel, D.; Adu, K.M.; Apiribu, F.; Bawontuo, V.; Adogboba, D.A.; Ali, K.T.; Mashamba-Thompson, T.P. Geographic accessibility to public health facilities providing tuberculosis testing services at point-of-care in the upper east region, Ghana. *BMC Public Health* **2019**, *19*, 718. [CrossRef] [PubMed]

13. Kuupiel, D.; Adu, K.M.; Bawontuo, V.; Mashamba-Thompson, T.P. Geographical Accessibility to District Hospitals/Medical Laboratories for Comprehensive Antenatal Point-of-Care Diagnostic Services in the Upper East Region, Ghana. *E. Clin. Med.* **2019**, *13*, 74–80. [CrossRef] [PubMed]
14. Ameyaw, E.K.; Kofinti, R.E.; Appiah, F. National health insurance subscription and maternal healthcare utilisation across mothers' wealth status in Ghana. *Health Econ. Rev.* **2017**, *7*, 16. [CrossRef] [PubMed]
15. Ghana Statistical Service, G.H.S.; ICF. Ghana Maternal Health Survey 2017: Key Findings. Available online: https://dhsprogram.com/pubs/pdf/SR251/SR251.pdf (accessed on 24 April 2019).
16. Asamoah, B.O.; Moussa, K.M.; Stafström, M.; Musinguzi, G. Distribution of causes of maternal mortality among different socio-demographic groups in Ghana; A descriptive study. *BMC Public Health* **2011**, *11*, 159. [CrossRef] [PubMed]
17. Der, E.M.; Moyer, C.; Gyasi, R.K.; Akosa, A.B.; Tettey, Y.; Akakpo, P.K.; Blankson, A.; Anim, J.T. Pregnancy Related Causes of Deaths in Ghana: A 5-Year Retrospective Study. *Ghana Med. J.* **2013**, *47*, 158–163. [PubMed]
18. Ministry of Health; Ghana Health Service. *Maternal Health Record Book*; Reproduction and Child Health, Ed.; Ministry of Health: Accra, Ghana, 2016; p. 4.
19. Republic of Ghana; Ghana Health Service. A guide for maternal and newborn care part one: Maternal care.
20. Kuupiel, D.; Tlou, B.; Bawontuo, V.; Mashamba-Thompson, T.P. Accessibility of pregnancy-related point-of-care diagnostic tests for maternal healthcare in rural primary healthcare facilities in Northern Ghana: A cross-sectional survey. *Heliyon* **2019**, *5*, e01236. [CrossRef] [PubMed]
21. World Health Organization. Second WHO Model List of Essential In Vitro Diagnostics. Available online: https://www.who.int/medical_devices/publications/Second_WHO_Model_List_of_Essential_In_Vitro_Diagnostics/en/ (accessed on 21 September 2019).
22. Becher, H.; Muller, O.; Jahn, A.; Gbangou, A.; Kynast-Wolf, G.; Kouyate, B. Risk factors of infant and child mortality in rural Burkina Faso. *Bull. World Health Organ.* **2004**, *82*, 265–273. [PubMed]
23. Anselin, L. Spatial Data Analysis with GIS: An Introduction to Application in the Social Sciences. Available online: https://escholarship.org/uc/item/58w157nm#main (accessed on 20 September 2019).
24. Environment Systems Research Institute. How Spatial Autocorrelation (Global Moran's I) works. Available online: https://pro.arcgis.com/en/pro-app/tool-reference/spatial-statistics/h-how-spatial-autocorrelation-moran-s-i-spatial-st.htm (accessed on 26 September 2019).
25. Brondeel, R.; Weill, A.; Thomas, F.; Chaix, B. Use of healthcare services in the residence and workplace neighbourhood: The effect of spatial accessibility to healthcare services. *Health Place* **2014**, *30*, 127–133. [CrossRef] [PubMed]
26. Ferguson, W.J.; Kemp, K.; Kost, G. Using a geographic information system to enhance patient access to point-of-care diagnostics in a limited-resource setting. *Int. J. Health Geogr.* **2016**, *15*, 10. [CrossRef] [PubMed]
27. Mitra, R.; Mishra, N.; Rath, G.P. Blood groups systems. *Indian J. Anaesth* **2014**, *58*, 524–528. [CrossRef] [PubMed]
28. Patel, A.; Waters, N. Using geographic information systems for health research. In *Application of Geographic Information Systems*; IntechOpen: London, UK, 2012.
29. Dangisso, M.H.; Datiko, D.G.; Lindtjorn, B. Accessibility to tuberculosis control services and tuberculosis programme performance in southern Ethiopia. *Glob. Health Action* **2015**, *8*, 29443. [CrossRef] [PubMed]
30. Kost, G. Theory, principles, and practice of optimizing point-of-care small-world networks. *Point Care* **2012**, *11*, 96–101. [CrossRef]

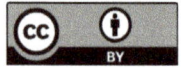

© 2019 by the authors. Licensee MDPI, Basel, Switzerland. This article is an open access article distributed under the terms and conditions of the Creative Commons Attribution (CC BY) license (http://creativecommons.org/licenses/by/4.0/).

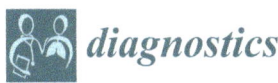

Article

Stakeholder Perceptions of Point-of-Care Ultrasound Implementation in Resource-Limited Settings

Anna M. Maw [1,*], Brittany Galvin [2], Ricardo Henri [2], Michael Yao [3], Bruno Exame [2], Michelle Fleshner [4], Meredith P. Fort [5] and Megan A. Morris [6]

1. Division of Hospital Medicine, University of Colorado, Aurora, CO 80045, USA
2. Alma Mater Hospital, Gros Morne 4210, Haiti; galvibr@gmail.com (B.G.); ricardsh93@yahoo.fr (R.H.); brunoexame@gmail.com (B.E.)
3. Division of Engineering and Applied Science, California Institute of Technology, Pasadena, CA 91125, USA; michael.yao@atriaconnect.org
4. Division of General Internal Medicine, University of Pittsburgh Medical Center, Pittsburgh, PA 15260, USA; fleshnerm@upmc.edu
5. Department of Health Systems, Management and Policy, Centers for American Indian and Alaska Native Health, Colorado School of Public Health, Aurora, CO 80045, USA; meredith.fort@cuanschutz.edu
6. Adult and Child Consortium for Health Outcomes Research and Delivery Science, University of Colorado School of Medicine, Aurora, CO 80045, USA; megan.a.morris@cuanschutz.edu
* Correspondence: anna.maw@cuanschutz.edu

Received: 30 September 2019; Accepted: 16 October 2019; Published: 18 October 2019

Abstract: Background: Nearly half of the world lacks access to diagnostic imaging. Point of care ultrasound (POCUS) is a versatile and relatively affordable imaging modality that offers promise as a means of bridging the radiology gap and improving care in low resource settings. Methods: We performed semi-structured interviews of key stakeholders at two diverse hospitals where POCUS implementation programs had recently been conducted: one in a rural private hospital in Haiti and the other in a public referral hospital in Malawi. Questions regarding the clinical utility of POCUS, as well as barriers and facilitators of its implementation, were asked of study participants. Using the Framework Method, analysis of interview transcripts was guided by the WHO ASSURED criteria for point of care diagnostics. Results: Fifteen stakeholders with diverse roles in POCUS implementation were interviewed. Interviewees from both sites considered POCUS a valuable diagnostic tool that improved clinical decisions. They perceived barriers to adequate training as one of the most important remaining barriers to POCUS implementation. Conclusions: In spite of the increasing affordability and portability of ultrasounds devices, there are still important barriers to the implementation of POCUS in resource-limited settings.

Keywords: point-of-care-ultrasound; ultrasound; implementation

1. Introduction

It has been estimated that approximately half of the world lacks access to even basic diagnostic imaging [1]. Among the factors responsible for what is termed the "radiology gap" is the high cost required to procure and maintain most radiology equipment and the specialized expertise of necessary personnel such as radiologists and technicians [2].

Studies show that 80–90% of imaging needs can be addressed with X-ray and ultrasound alone [3,4]. Ultrasound is particularly versatile and is the least expensive of all imaging modalities [2]. Common applications of ultrasound that routinely change management decisions in low resource settings [5,6] include the diagnosis of pneumonia, extrapulmonary tuberculosis, parasitic infections, rheumatic heart disease, and ectopic pregnancy [7–9]. In addition, as noncommunicable diseases such as heart disease become more prevalent in low- and middle-income countries, so too does the utility of ultrasound in these settings [10].

Recognizing ultrasound as the most promising modality to bridge the radiology gap, the World Health Organization (WHO) published a series of documents beginning in the 1990s designed to facilitate the implementation of ultrasound more broadly [11,12]. At that time, the WHO warned that operator training was one of the biggest barriers to appropriate implementation.

Over the last 20 years, ultrasound has become even more portable and much less costly, allowing for the development of a new practice called point-of-care ultrasound (POCUS) [13], in which images are acquired and interpreted by the treating clinician at the bedside. POCUS is a growing field in Europe and the United States, with emerging evidence that it improves time to diagnosis and decreases cost in high-resource settings [14,15]. In contrast to consultative ultrasound, which is technician-performed and interpreted by a radiologist, POCUS answers focused diagnostic questions using easily performed techniques that can be quickly interpreted at the bedside. Because POCUS addresses focused questions and is not a comprehensive evaluation of an organ system, image acquisition and interpretation are easier to master than traditional consultative ultrasound. This aspect of POCUS reduces one of the remaining significant barriers to ultrasound's widespread use in resource-limited settings: extensive training.

The reduced price of hand-held ultrasound machines, which cost approximately 10,000 USD in contrast to standard ultrasound machines which are about 50,000 USD [16], makes POCUS a particularly good fit for resource-limited settings, as does its immediate availability of results and lack of reliance on additional infrastructure and personnel (e.g., technicians, radiologists, and laboratories). Continued improvements in cost, portability, and battery life all will all serve to reduce barriers to its implementation over time. Given the dynamic nature of factors that influence the implementation of POCUS and the expanding applications of its use, the purpose of this study is to determine the current barriers and facilitators of its implementation in low-resource settings.

2. Materials and Methods

2.1. Study Sample and Setting

The Institutional Review Board at University of Colorado deemed this study not Human Subjects research. We obtained written consent from all participants prior to their interview. We interviewed key stakeholders from 2 diverse hospital settings in which POCUS implementation programs had recently been conducted. One site was in a private rural 60 bed hospital in Haiti and the other was an 800 bed referral hospital in Malawi. Key stakeholders from both sites were interviewed as part of the study. We defined a key stakeholder as an individual who in some way influences the implementation of POCUS. The following types of stakeholders were included in the study: program initiators (individuals who established the POCUS implementation program), POCUS instructors, hospital administrators, provider trainees, and local physician leaders.

2.2. Data Collection

Data for this study were collected between July 2019 and September 2019. The WHO ASSURED criteria [17] (Table 1) were used to shape the interview guide, data coding and analysis. These criteria were developed by the WHO Sexually Transmitted Diseases Diagnostics Initiative to describe the characteristics of the perfect point-of-care diagnostic test in resource-limited settings. However, we feel it outlines important considerations for any type of diagnostic test and highlights many of the reasons why POCUS is uniquely positioned to be the most effective imaging modality for low-resource settings.

Table 1. WHO ASSURED Criteria.

Affordable (Affordable to the Communities Who Need It)
Sensitive
Specific
User-Friendly (Simple to perform requiring minimal training)
Rapid and Robust (Quick results that enable treatment on the first visit)
Equipment-free (minimal reliance on technological infrastructure)
Delivered (Ability to be delivered to those who need it; portable)

Semistructured interviews were conducted with key stakeholders to assess their perspective on point of care ultrasound implementation in their local setting and more broadly. Interviews were conducted by phone and in person. Some interviews were conducted in English and some in Creole, depending on the language spoken by the interviewee. Those conducted in English were conducted by AMM. Those conducted in Creole were performed by BG, who both conducted the interviews and translated answers into English during the interview. Interviews were conducted until thematic saturation was reached: when no additional themes were immerging from the interviews. All interviews were conducted using the same interview guide (see Supplementary Materials).

2.3. Data Entry and Analysis

The interviews were audio recorded and transcribed verbatim. We used a framework analysis [18] and a largely deductive approach. Our coding framework was informed by the WHO ASSURED criteria. We were also open to new themes that may have arisen inductively from the data. Our coding process was guided by consensus qualitative research methods [19]. The consensus research approach has the following features: data were collected through open-ended questions in semi-structured interviews, interviews were analyzed to achieve consensus of at least 2 analysts, an outside auditor (a qualitative expert not integrally involved in the study) supervised the process to help maximize the validity of the findings, thematic content analysis was performed by AMM, study site leaders BG (Haiti) and MF (Malawi) reviewed the categorization of themes obtained from stakeholders at their respective sites to ensure the validity of the analysis, and MAM acted as the qualitative expert supervising the analysis.

Patterns of POCUS implementation facilitators and barriers were identified from participants' interviews. First, participants' responses were coded into framework categories, which were then grouped into themes.

3. Results

A total of 15 interviews were conducted by key stakeholders (Table 2) at two sites located in a small private rural hospital in Haiti and a large public referral hospital in Malawi. Interview length ranged from 20 to 45 min.

Table 2. Stakeholder interviewees and their role in POCUS implementation.

Type of Stakeholder	Description of Stakeholders
2 Program Founders	Both individuals were from the United States: 1 began the implementation program in Haiti and the other initiated the program in Malawi.
3 Instructors	All 3 were physicians from the United States with expertise in POCUS: 1 internist who taught in Haiti and 2 medical residents who taught in Malawi.
8 Trainees	All were local providers: 1 nurse practitioner, 2 residents, 1 internist, and 1 gynecologist who worked in Haiti, and 2 registrars and 1 intern who worked in Malawi.
2 Hospital Administrators	Both were associated with the site in Haiti.

The study aimed to understand factors that may affect the implementation and sustainability of POCUS in low-resource settings. Guided by the WHO ASSURED criteria for point-of-care diagnostics in resource limited settings, core themes were identified (Table 3).

Table 3. Themes identified from interview data.

Framework Domain	Subthemes	Subtheme by Site
Affordability	Cost and Cost Saving	
	cost of machines	Haiti and Malawi
		it was much easier to obtain machines by external funders than in the past
	cost of training	Haiti and Malawi
		local providers were unable to pay the cost of classes
	cost saving to patient	Haiti
		availability of POCUS allowed patients to be diagnosed locally instead of having to travel to the referral hospital
		Malawi
		POCUS exams did not affect cost to the patient as all care was free
	cost savings to hospital	Haiti
		availability of POCUS allowed patients who would normally be referred to another hospital, to be diagnosed locally which in turn allowed them to purchase care and medications locally
		Malawi
		POCUS did not affect cost or cost savings to the hospital
Accuracy	greatly improved diagnosis and management	Haiti and Malawi
		POCUS improved accuracy for many diagnoses at both hospitals, expediating appropriate treatment and making procedures safer
User-friendly	language barrier	Haiti
		language barrier between instructors and local providers was a barrier to training
		Malawi
		language was not a barrier in Malawi as both instructors and local providers spoke English
	requires significant training	Haiti and Malawi
		the amount of time required for training was considered an important barrier at both sites
	lack of continuity of staff	Haiti and Malawi
		lack of clinician continuity at both sites created a barrier to training as there was no expert consistently available to teach others

Table 3. *Cont.*

Framework Domain	Subthemes	Subtheme by Site
Rapid and Robust	greatly decreased time to imaging	*Haiti*
		no consultative ultrasound was available, therefore POCUS improved time to diagnosis as because patients did not have to travel to a referral hospital for an ultrasound
		Malawi
		POCUS allowed for more rapid diagnosis as there was a long wait for X-rays and consultative ultrasound
Equipment-free	no expertise to fix hand-held ultrasound locally	*Haiti and Malawi*
		concerns were expressed regarding what to do if a machine broke because there is no local expert to fix a hand-held ultrasound
	loss of hand-held ultrasound.	*Haiti and Malawi*
		concerns were expressed about the likelihood of a hand-held ultrasound being lost given its small size
Delivered	diagnosis in rural locations.	*Haiti*
		POCUS allowed patients to be diagnosed in a rural hospital setting without requiring travel to another larger hospital
	diagnosis of patients too ill to travel	*Malawi*
		POCUS allowed patients that could not physically be moved to radiology department to be diagnosed at referral hospital.
		POCUS also allowed diagnosis via home visits when patients were not able to travel to the hospital
Inductive Themes	development of local experts	*Haiti and Malawi*
		study participants recommended focusing resources on the development of local clinicians so that they can assume the role of local experts and can train other local clinicians
	remote learning technology	*Haiti and Malawi*
		the expense and unreliability of the internet limited access to remote learning

3.1. Affordability

The costs associated with several aspects of implementation were considered barriers. Expenditures included costs related to adequate accessibility to machines and training.

In addition, interviewees in Haiti expressed the potential of cost-savings to both the patients and hospital associated with ultrasound as it allowed for local diagnosis and treatment rather than referral to a larger facility.

3.1.1. Cost Related to Machines

Stakeholders expressed that although machines were more accessible than they had been previously, this cost was still considered a barrier to implementation. This was the case in part because even if providers had received training in the past, if there was no machine in their current practice setting they would not be able to maintain their skill.

> "After the people who are training the doctors leave, we need to be sure that there are ultrasound machines available for everyone to practice. Even if there are ultrasounds at some hospitals, doctors often take different jobs and if those ultrasounds aren't available at all hospitals then everything that the doctor learned they might forget because they don't have the ultrasound available to them. Therefore, they would lose this skill."

3.1.2. Cost Related to Training

The cost related to training was also perceived as a significant barrier to implementation.

> "It was the gynecologist we had on staff who said, 'You know, I've always wanted to go to a more formal ultrasound program, but when I looked at them, they were like 1,500, 2,500 U.S. dollars.' He goes, 'I can't afford that'." (Haiti)

3.1.3. Cost to the Patient

Interviewees associated with the Haiti site felt POCUS improved cost from the perspective of the patients because it allowed them to receive a diagnosis locally thereby avoiding both the expense of travel to a referral hospital and the cost of a consultative ultrasound once there.

> "Advantage was for patients because they used to have to travel and spend a lot of money to be able to have ultrasound diagnostics in other locations. Now that we have the diagnosis here, they don't have to travel and they don't have to pay a fee for the diagnostics." (Haiti)

In contrast, in Malawi, because it was a public hospital, there was no additional cost to the patients because all care was free.

> "The hospital that I work at is a public hospital so everything is included. For things that are able to be done at the public hospital it's not an issue . . . . for the purposes of the ultrasounds, and the X-rays, they're not charged anything." (Malawi)

3.1.4. Revenue Generation for the Hospital

Interviewees in Haiti also noted that being able to offer ultrasound may generate revenue for the hospital because when they are able to receive a diagnosis locally, they can remain at the hospital for treatment.

> "If we could increase the utilization of the service in the hospital it would be a huge benefit because we would become more competent in ultrasound and we could take on more patients . . . . therefore, keeping more patients in the hospital. Not having to refer them. And also, the hospital would be able to make more money because we are not having to send people away." (Haiti)

3.2. Accuracy (Sensitivity and Specificity)

All interviewees from both sites believed POCUS improved diagnosis and management decisions significantly.

> "Actually I think that the Point of Care Ultrasound is very, very important in taking care of the patient particularly in the resource limited settings. We don't really have access to imaging modalities

like MRI, CT. With ultrasound we can get a lot of information for most parts of the body. You can scan the lungs, you can scan the heart, you can scan the abdomen, you can scan pretty much everywhere. I think that this is actually a very helpful tool that would help improving healthcare in settings like this." (Haiti)

"We are looking at a lot of people being misdiagnosed. We kind of have a lot of deaths that may be would have been averted if we'd have really known what was happening." (Malawi)

"Most people here do paras and thoras completely blind. So training them to use POCUS to do procedures more safely would be another big benefit." (Malawi)

3.3. User-Friendly

Once proficient, trainees felt POCUS exams were quick and easy to perform. However, all interviewees felt that adequate training was currently an important barrier to use. Subthemes included (1) language barriers between trainees and instructors; (2) limited time for trainees to attend trainings when offered because of clinical responsibilities; (3) lack of continuity of staff who have been trained.

3.3.1. Language

Interviewees in Haiti reported language as a barrier to training, in that the majority of instructors spoke English but almost all of the trainees spoke Creole and French. Language was not reported as a barrier by stakeholders from the hospital in Malawi where the instructors and trainees all spoke English.

"One challenge was for the foreigners who came to teach the lesson. We don't speak the same language, so there was a language difficulty." (Haiti)

3.3.2. Time to Attend Trainings

Interviewees at both sites reported that clinical responsibilities were an important barrier to attending training sessions when offered.

"The biggest challenge was that we were trying to take care of the patients at the same time as learning because we still had a role at the hospital. We didn't have time off." (Haiti)

"In general, our medical department right now is super short-staffed and so the interns are really overworked. So the time it takes to train is another big barrier." (Malawi)

3.3.3. Lack of Clinician Continuity

Interviewees at both sites reported lack of clinician continuity was an important barrier to implementation and sustainability.

"So it's a little bit harder because if we were to train them, then they're gone in three months. So they're not a sustainable part of the process." (Malawi)

"They come and go now and then, and this is actually another challenge. Some of the doctors trained have already left the hospital." (Haiti)

3.4. Rapid and Robust

Interviewees expressed that one of the important benefits of POCUS is that results are immediately available. This was an important advantage at the rural hospital in Haiti, where there was no consultative ultrasound available and patients were often unable to return for test results. It was important at the referral hospital in Malawi as well because there were such long waits for consultative ultrasound performed by radiology.

"The advantages are tremendous because so often our X-ray machine isn't working, and/or it's a terrible X-ray machine, the images aren't clear. Plus we're so limited in referral, if you're in the States, if you have a patient who is injured, even if they're not at one hospital, you can quickly transfer them to another hospital. In Haiti it's not so much the case. In addition to the cost of care can be astronomical. So free point of care testing that can be rapid, on the spot is a huge advantage for diagnosis and treatment." (Haiti)

"If maybe most of the clinicians, can be trained on how to use an ultrasound, it'll be far better, because instead of sending the patient to radiology they can be doing it on their own. Because most of the time it will be like, 'Okay, it'll be done like in the next three days, because there a lot of patients that are waiting.'" (Malawi)

3.5. Equipment-Free

Interviewees expressed that the hand-held ultrasounds were easier to maintain than other forms of radiology (X-ray, commuted tomography, and consultative ultrasound). Interestingly, interviewees related times that POCUS findings were useful as surrogates for laboratory results because basic labs were not reliably available at either site. Due to its small size, loss of the hand-held ultrasound was more of a concern than need for repair or maintenance. However, although neither site reported an instance in which a hand-held ultrasound had required maintenance or repair, interviewees expressed concern that there was no local technician to repair it should the need arise.

"I think one of the biggest challenges with respect to the ultrasound and with respect to a lot of other things is that equipment tends to walk off. And so I think in terms of buy-in, there needs to be somebody who's kind of the gatekeeper and keeps the device from disappearing." (Malawi)

"And if there's a problem with the equipment, who's qualified to repair it or to troubleshoot? Because we don't have technicians of that nature available in Haiti." (Haiti)

3.6. Delivered

Interviewees at both sites reported that POCUS was extremely portable, all but eliminating time and resources spent on delivery and installation which are important barriers to implementation with other radiologic modalities [2]. Stakeholders at the Haiti site reported having a hand-held device available allowed for diagnosis locally instead of needing to refer patients to a larger hospital with consultative ultrasound or other imaging modalities. Stakeholders at the site reported being able to obtain imaging on patients too sick to come to the hospital via home visits and those in the hospital but too sick to travel to radiology.

"For my other job ... they do home visits. So there have been a couple times that there are people who can't come to clinic because of whatever, because they've had a stroke or et cetera. There've been a couple times that I've gone out with residents and taken the ultrasound with me and that is really, really useful. So I mean, I think that there would be a real benefit to that." (Malawi)

"Now that it's in the hospital, they don't even have to leave the hospital. Therefore, they're not having to spend this money and have more money to buy the medicine that they need. Basically, they can get all the care that they need in one place inside of the hospital." (Haiti)

3.7. Inductive Themes

3.7.1. Development and Support of Local Experts

One inductive theme that emerged from stakeholders in both Haiti and Malawi was a recommendation to support a few local providers to undergo significant training in POCUS and then offer them support to train other local providers.

"So would there have been a possibility of appointing one physician and maybe giving them an extra stipend to encourage them, or sign a contract saying 'Hey, we're going to train you in this. This is your three year contract and these are the objectives of hiring you as this. Not only are you going to see patients, but you're going to be the lead for this and you're responsible to train other physicians as they come in.' So there is, even if we have turnover, there is a plan to engage new physicians as we bring them aboard." (Haiti)

"Getting the Registrars to be excited about POCUS because they're the one who will really be doing it. They're the ones that teach the interns, they're the ones who teach the med students. Getting a few of them trained and then going from there would be the best strategy. ... The barrier is that they get paid virtually nothing so they all end up basically taking second jobs at private hospitals or private clinics and then end up not being at work as much. ... I think if we were able to provide one or two people with extra money to do POCUS training and that was their incentive, I think that would be huge." (Malawi)

3.7.2. Remote Learning Technology

Another inductive theme that emerged was the potential but current limitations of the internet as a means of providing remote learning opportunities and addressing the barrier of training without local experts available.

"We did develop this way of uploading all of our images to Google Drive and then creating a log and a spreadsheet of logging all of our images. Basically 250 images QA'd by people from the states. So, the goal ultimately would be to do that with local providers and I think it would work but there's a few big barriers. The biggest of which is paying. We had to use data, straight phone data for it and it probably cost like $100 over the course of two months. Which isn't a lot here but it's not a sustainable thing for them to do. So that's kind of a challenge." (Malawi)

"Actually it is a challenge, in such limited settings, even the Internet, we had the devices, they had an integrated software called 'React' that allows remote education, but we couldn't use it properly because of the Internet. We had Internet access at the hospital, but it was a very low speed. We couldn't really use it. Internet access as well is a barrier. Like with Internet we could have been able to do remote education, it would have been much easier to do it." (Haiti)

4. Discussion

To our knowledge, this is the first study to explore the barriers and facilitators of POCUS implementation in resource-limited settings using qualitative methods. Our findings demonstrate the perceived clinical utility of POCUS, as well as the remaining barriers to implementation and sustainability. All stakeholders expressed the belief that POCUS had the potential to greatly improve management decisions and patient care but felt that the cost and time required for training were major barriers to implementation. Other barriers identified by study participants included the lack of continuity of providers at each site that would allow retention of an institutional expert to provide longitudinal mentorship as well as curriculum development and implementation which would be required for trainees to attain competency. Additional barriers included equipment maintenance and accessibility. This finding is consistent with other studies on this topic [20]. Interviewees also reported the local internet services were currently too slow, unreliable, or expensive to use effectively for remote learning. However, it is important to note that given the pace of advances in both remote learning technology and artificial intelligence applications [21], the former allowing for accelerated training and the later offering automated image interpretation, a swift decline in training as a barrier to POCUS implementation is expected.

Stakeholders at both sites recommended focusing resources on the training of a small number of local providers that could then become educators for their region, which would address many of the barriers expressed. This approach would provide: (1) longitudinal mentoring to other local providers; (2) someone who would be accountable for maintaining equipment; (3) elimination of language barriers between instructor and learner; and (4) reduce the cost related to providing training (e.g., resources that would otherwise be invested in travel and time of nonlocal experts may instead be invested into local champions).

Limitations

There are several important limitations to our study. The first is that we only interviewed stakeholders associated with two POCUS implementation program sites. This may limit the generalizability of our results. However, the sites were diverse clinical environments, one a small rural private hospital and the other a large public referral hospital, located in different countries. Additionally, the barriers that emerged as themes included the cost of the machines, language barriers, and lack of continuity of experts which would be expected to apply to many low-resource settings, suggesting many of our findings are to some extent generalizable. The study also would have been improved by gaining a broader healthcare system perspective by interviewing people within the Ministry of Health in each of the countries represented to determine whether they consider POCUS implementation worth investing in. Additionally, because a third of the study participants and most of research team is from the United States it is possible that we failed to capture all relevant themes accurately due to cultural bias. Finally, some of our interviews were done by phone as opposed to in-person which may have resulted in loss of contextual or nonverbal information. However, given the subject matter, which is of a relatively concrete and unsensitive nature, we feel it is unlikely this greatly influenced the themes that emerged.

5. Conclusions

POCUS is considered a highly effective diagnostic tool that improves patient care by all stakeholders interviewed. Although more affordable, the cost of machines is still a barrier to implementation of POCUS, though the expense and time required for optimal training of local providers seems to be the most important current barrier. Our findings highlight the remaining barriers to implementation as well as offer potential strategies to overcome them.

Supplementary Materials: The following are available online at http://www.mdpi.com/2075-4418/9/4/153/s1: Interview Guide.

Author Contributions: Study conceptualization, A.M.M., M.P.F., M.A.M.; methodology, M.A.M.; data collection A.M.M, B.G.; writing—original draft preparation, A.M.M.; writing—review and editing, M.Y., R.H., B.E., B.G., M.F., M.P.F., M.A.M.; supervision, M.A.M.

Funding: This research received no external funding.

Acknowledgments: The authors would like to thank Gordy Johnson and Sr Jacqueline Picard without whom this manuscript would not have been possible.

Conflicts of Interest: The authors declare no conflict of interest.

References

1. Mollura, D.J.; Soroosh, G.; Culp, M.P.; RAD-AID Conference Writing Group. 2016 RAD-AID Conference on International Radiology for Developing Countries: Gaps, Growth, and United Nations Sustainable Development Goals. *J. Am. Coll. Radiol.* **2017**, *14*, 841–847. [CrossRef] [PubMed]
2. Mollura, D.L.; Lungren, M.P. *Radiology in Global Health*; Springer: Cham, Switzerland, 2019.
3. Ostensen, H.; Volodin, V. Diagnostic imaging in developing countries: Considerations for improvement. *Eur. Radiol.* **2000**, *10*, S397–S398. [CrossRef] [PubMed]
4. Maru, D.S.; Schwarz, R.; Jason, A.; Basu, S.; Sharma, A.; Moore, C. Turning a blind eye: The mobilization of radiology services in resource-poor regions. *Glob. Health* **2010**, *6*, 18. [CrossRef] [PubMed]

5. Becker, D.M.; Tafoya, C.A.; Becker, S.L.; Kruger, G.H.; Tafoya, M.J.; Becker, T.K. The use of portable ultrasound devices in low- and middle-income countries: A systematic review of the literature. *Trop. Med. Int. Health* **2016**, *21*, 294–311. [CrossRef] [PubMed]
6. Reynolds, T.A.; Amato, S.; Kulola, I.; Chen, C.J.; Mfinanga, J.; Sawe, H.R. Impact of point-of-care ultrasound on clinical decision-making at an urban emergency department in Tanzania. *PLoS ONE* **2018**, *13*, e0194774. [CrossRef] [PubMed]
7. Saxena, A. Rheumatic heart disease screening by "point-of-care" echocardiography: An acceptable alternative in resource limited settings? *Transl. Pediatr.* **2015**, *4*, 210–213. [CrossRef] [PubMed]
8. Fentress, M.; Heyne, T.F.; Barron, K.R.; Jayasekera, N. Point-of-Care Ultrasound in Resource-Limited Settings: Common Applications. *South. Med. J.* **2018**, *111*, 424–433. [CrossRef] [PubMed]
9. Groen, R.S.; Leow, J.J.; Sadasivam, V.; Kushner, A.L. Review: Indications for ultrasound use in low- and middle-income countries. *Trop. Med. Int. Health* **2011**, *16*, 1525–1535. [CrossRef] [PubMed]
10. Mehta, M.; Jacobson, T.; Peters, D.; Le, E.; Chadderdon, S.; Allen, A.J.; Caughey, A.B.; Kaul, S. Handheld ultrasound versus physical examination in patients referred for transthoracic echocardiography for a suspected cardiac condition. *JACC Cardiovasc. Imaging* **2014**, *7*, 983–990. [CrossRef] [PubMed]
11. Goldberg, B.B. Training in diagnostic ultrasound: Essentials, principles and standards. Report of a WHO Study Group. *World Health Organ. Tech. Rep. Ser.* **1998**, *875*, i-46.
12. Lutz, H.; Buscarini, E.; Mirk, P. *Manuel of Diagnostic Ultrasound*, 2nd ed.; WHO: Geneva, Switerland, 2013; Volume 1.
13. Soni, N.; Arntfield, R.; Kory, P. *Point of Care Ultrasound*; Elsevier: Philadelphia, PA, USA, 2019; p. 1.
14. Zanobetti, M.; Scorpiniti, M.; Gigli, C.; Nazerian, P.; Vanni, S.; Innocenti, F.; Stefanone, V.T.; Savinelli, C.; Coppa, A.; Bigiarini, S.; et al. Point-of-Care Ultrasonography for Evaluation of Acute Dyspnea in the ED. *Chest* **2017**, *151*, 1295–1301. [CrossRef] [PubMed]
15. Smallwood, N.; Dachsel, M. Point-of-care ultrasound (POCUS): Unnecessary gadgetry or evidence-based medicine? *Clin. Med. (Lond)* **2018**, *18*, 219–224. [CrossRef] [PubMed]
16. Tse, K.H.; Luk, W.H.; Lam, M.C. Pocket-sized versus standard ultrasound machines in abdominal imaging. *Singap. Med. J.* **2014**, *55*, 325–333. [CrossRef] [PubMed]
17. Mabey, D.; Peeling, R.W.; Ustianowski, A.; Perkins, M.D. Diagnostics for the developing world. *Nat. Rev. Microbiol.* **2004**, *2*, 231–240. [CrossRef] [PubMed]
18. Gale, N.K.; Heath, G.; Cameron, E.; Rashid, S.; Redwood, S. Using the framework method for the analysis of qualitative data in multi-disciplinary health research. *BMC Med. Res. Methodol.* **2013**, *13*, 117. [CrossRef] [PubMed]
19. Hill, C.E.; Knox, S.; Thompson, B.J.; Williams, E.N.; Hess, S.A.; Ladany, N. Consensual qualitative research: An update. *J. Couns. Psychol.* **2005**, *52*, 196–205. [CrossRef]
20. Shah, S.; Bellows, B.A.; Adedipe, A.A.; Totten, J.E.; Backlund, B.H.; Sajed, D. Perceived barriers in the use of ultrasound in developing countries. *Crit. Ultrasound J.* **2015**, *7*, 28. [CrossRef]
21. Shokoohi, H.; LeSaux, M.A.; Roohani, Y.H.; Liteplo, A.; Huang, C.; Blaivas, M. Enhanced Point-of-Care Ultrasound Applications by Integrating Automated Feature-Learning Systems Using Deep Learning. *J. Ultrasound Med.* **2019**, *38*, 1887–1897. [CrossRef]

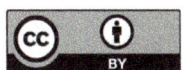

© 2019 by the authors. Licensee MDPI, Basel, Switzerland. This article is an open access article distributed under the terms and conditions of the Creative Commons Attribution (CC BY) license (http://creativecommons.org/licenses/by/4.0/).

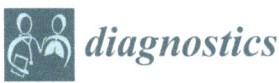

Article

Feasibility Evaluation of Commercially Available Video Conferencing Devices to Technically Direct Untrained Nonmedical Personnel to Perform a Rapid Trauma Ultrasound Examination

Davinder Ramsingh [1,*], Michael Ma [2], Danny Quy Le [3], Warren Davis [4], Mark Ringer [5], Briahnna Austin [1] and Cameron Ricks [2]

1. Department of Anesthesiology, Loma Linda University Health, 11234 Anderson St. MC-2532, Loma Linda, CA 92354, USA; BRAustin@llu.edu
2. Department of Anesthesiology, UCI Medical Center, Orange, CA 92868, USA; ma.michael@gmail.com (M.M.); cricks@uci.edu (C.R.)
3. David Geffen School of Medicine at UCLA, Los Angeles, CA 90095, USA; dannyle097@gmail.com
4. Department of Anesthesiology, St. Joseph Medical Center, 7601 Osler Drive, Towson, MD 21204, USA; wardav@gmail.com
5. Loma Linda University School of Medicine, Loma Linda, CA 92350, USA; mringer@llu.edu
* Correspondence: dramsingh@llu.edu

Received: 1 October 2019; Accepted: 11 November 2019; Published: 14 November 2019

Abstract: Introduction: Point-of-care ultrasound (POCUS) is a rapidly expanding discipline that has proven to be a valuable modality in the hospital setting. Recent evidence has demonstrated the utility of commercially available video conferencing technologies, namely, FaceTime (Apple Inc, Cupertino, CA, USA) and Google Glass (Google Inc, Mountain View, CA, USA), to allow an expert POCUS examiner to remotely guide a novice medical professional. However, few studies have evaluated the ability to use these teleultrasound technologies to guide a nonmedical novice to perform an acute care POCUS examination for cardiac, pulmonary, and abdominal assessments. Additionally, few studies have shown the ability of a POCUS-trained cardiac anesthesiologist to perform the role of an expert instructor. This study sought to evaluate the ability of a POCUS-trained anesthesiologist to remotely guide a nonmedically trained participant to perform an acute care POCUS examination. **Methods:** A total of 21 nonmedically trained undergraduate students who had no prior ultrasound experience were recruited to perform a three-part ultrasound examination on a standardized patient with the guidance of a remote expert who was a POCUS-trained cardiac anesthesiologist. The examination included the following acute care POCUS topics: (1) cardiac function via parasternal long/short axis views, (2) pneumothorax assessment via pleural sliding exam via anterior lung views, and (3) abdominal free fluid exam via right upper quadrant abdominal view. Each examiner was given a handout with static images of probe placement and actual ultrasound images for the three views. After a brief 8 min tutorial on the teleultrasound technologies, a connection was established with the expert, and they were guided through the acute care POCUS exam. Each view was deemed to be complete when the expert sonographer was satisfied with the obtained image or if the expert sonographer determined that the image could not be obtained after 5 min. Image quality was scored on a previously validated 0 to 4 grading scale. The entire session was recorded, and the image quality was scored during the exam by the remote expert instructor as well as by a separate POCUS-trained, blinded expert anesthesiologist. **Results:** A total of 21 subjects completed the study. The average total time for the exam was 8.5 min (standard deviation = 4.6). A comparison between the live expert examiner and the blinded postexam reviewer showed a 100% agreement between image interpretations. A review of the exams rated as three or higher demonstrated that 87% of abdominal, 90% of cardiac, and 95% of pulmonary exams achieved this level of image quality. A satisfaction survey of the novice users demonstrated higher ease of following commands for the cardiac and pulmonary exams compared to the abdominal exam. **Conclusions:** The results from this pilot study demonstrate that nonmedically trained individuals can be guided to complete a relevant ultrasound examination within a short period. Further evaluation of using telemedicine technologies to promote POCUS should be evaluated.

Keywords: point-of-care ultrasound; telemedicine; medical education

1. Introduction

Historically, the development of technology in medicine has more often been at the burden of higher costs. Indeed, recent reports suggest that, despite its increasing use, the cost of medical technology is not decreasing [1]. However, two areas in medicine in which this has been disproven are the categories of telemedicine and portable ultrasound.

Early ultrasound devices were large and often confined to hospital facilities that support imaging laboratories (cardiology, radiology, and obstetrics). With recent advances in ultrasound technology, however, these devices have become more portable, smaller, cheaper, and usable at the patient's bedside [2]. Indeed, point-of-care ultrasound (POCUS) has been identified as the most rapidly growing sector in medical ultrasound imaging, with handheld devices costing approximately 1/20th the price of 10 years ago (from $40,000 + to $2000) [3]. In addition, ultrasound provides the particular benefit of a significantly lower level of harm compared to other medical imaging modalities [4].

Point-of-care ultrasound refers to the use of portable ultrasonography at the patient's bedside for diagnostic and therapeutic purposes [5]. POCUS has been proven to serve a vital role in the rapid assessment of a patient's cardiac, pulmonary, hemodynamic, vascular, neurologic, and gastrointestinal status [4,6–8]. Additionally, the application of POCUS continues to broaden as its usefulness and efficiency are shown to be greater than alternative imaging [4,9]. While the clinical utility of POCUS is rapidly expanding, the majority of the evidence supports its utility by skilled practitioners with advanced medical training. However, with innovations in POCUS devices described above, the possibility of using this technology in settings where skilled practitioners are not available becomes more feasible. Indeed, the barrier to using POCUS in resource-limited settings may be secondary to a lack of education rather than the availability of equipment.

The area of telemedicine has also undergone a similar transformation to POCUS over recent years. Telemedicine is defined as the use of medical information exchanged from one site to another via electronic communications to improve patients' health status. The incorporation of consumer-level products has significantly reduced costs and has allowed this topic to become much more mainstream [10]. Indeed, consumer devices are demonstrating adequate capability for performing remote patient examinations, with continued improvements each year [10]. Furthermore, these technologies have advanced to allow hands-free video communication, with the remote viewer having a point-of-view (POV) perspective [11]. This innovation opens up new possibilities for application toward patient care.

Recently, consumer-available wearable technologies, such as Google Glass (GG; Mountain View, CA, USA), and routine video conferencing smartphone devices, such as Apple iPhone (Cupertino, CA, USA), have demonstrated utility in healthcare. The GG POV technology has demonstrated utility for improving intraoperative communication and documentation as well as surgical training [12]. The use of the FaceTime (FT) video conferencing technology from iPhone has demonstrated utility across a wide area of telemedicine applications. An abbreviated review demonstrated FT-supported telemedicine to be useful for primary care patient evaluation [13], dermatology evaluation [14], and management in the intensive care unit [15] as well as for improving the education of ultrasound-guided anesthetic procedures [16] and even airway management [17].

The integration of these two rapidly advancing areas (POCUS and telemedicine) has been explored. Recent evidence has demonstrated the ability of a POCUS expert physician to guide a nonphysician hospital staff member to perform a POCUS exam via consumer-available teleconference equipment [9]. This same research group also demonstrated the ability of FT technology to transfer ultrasound images without clinically significant quality degradation [18]. Moreover, the use of FT communication between an intensivist team at a tertiary care center and nonphysician healthcare providers in a low-income country demonstrated the ability to successfully educate about POCUS image acquisition techniques as well allow appropriate image quality for remote clinical interpretation [10]. Additionally, Zennaro et al. demonstrated a high degree of agreement between ultrasound exams performed by pediatricians who were guided remotely by radiologists and ultrasound exams performed by radiologists in person [19]. Similar results were found for the use of ultrasound with telemedicine (teleultrasound) for remote guidance between onsite resident physicians and remote expert mentors for the diagnosis of pediatric acute appendicitis [20]. Recently, the incorporation of augmented reality has also demonstrated utility for remote ultrasound guidance [21]. Finally, the development of a teleultrasound system that allows an expert to perform an ultrasound exam remotely via a robotic system has also demonstrated clinical utility [22].

While the utilization of teleultrasound has rapidly increased across many specialties for in-hospital patient care, far less has been explored for the use of POCUS technology to facilitate the management of patients in the out-of-hospital setting. Moreover, while the efficacy of teleultrasound between medical personnel has demonstrated patient benefit, there is much less evidence on the utility of implementing teleultrasound between a POCUS-trained physician and a person without medical training. Given the advancements in teleultrasound technology, there may be a potential to use these devices in resource-limited areas in which significant medical training is not available.

This scenario demonstrates the utility of evaluating the use of a low-cost teleultrasound system to guide nonmedical personnel to perform POCUS exams remotely. This pilot study sought to evaluate the ability of a POCUS-trained physician to remotely guide nonmedical personnel to perform an acute cardiac, pulmonary, and abdominal POCUS exam using consumer-available communication devices, namely, FT and GG. Specifically, this blinded study sought to evaluate the quality of images captured by untrained, nonmedical, tele-ultrasound-guided sonographers in comparison to the quality of images performed by an expert sonographer.

2. Methods

2.1. Study Design

This prospective, educational intervention study was approved by the Institutional Review Board (IRB # # 2014-1014) at the University of California—Irvine, Orange CA on 21 February 2014.

2.2. Population and Setting

Subjects were undergraduate students at the University of California, Irvine, who voluntarily consented to participate and who confirmed to having no medical ultrasound training.

2.3. Point-of-Care Ultrasound Exam

A previously validated point-of-care ultrasound was designed for the assessment of cardiovascular trauma (ACT) and included (1) cardiac evaluation via parasternal long and short-axis views, (2) pulmonary evaluation for pneumothorax via anterior lung sliding evaluation, and (3) abdominal free fluid evaluation via right upper quadrant scan (Figure 1) [23]. A high-frequency transducer (12 mHz) was used for pulmonary evaluation, and a low-frequency (2–5 mHz) transducer was used for cardiac and abdominal evaluation.

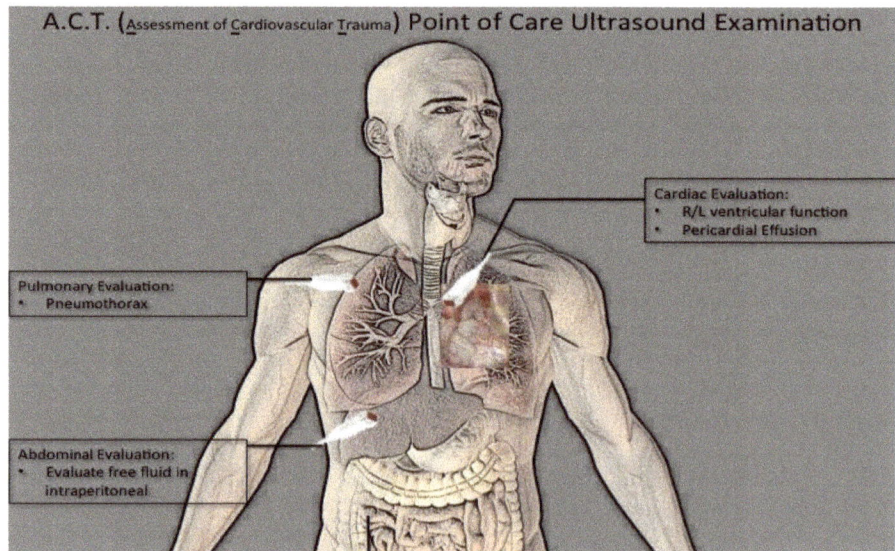

Figure 1. Focused ultrasound examination for assessment of cardiovascular trauma.

2.4. Experimental Protocol

After consent, participants received an 8 min tutorial on the following: ultrasound equipment (how to switch ultrasound probes, adjust depth, adjust gain, and locate the probe indicator), Google Glass (how to wear and connect audio), and iPhone FT video conferencing technology. The subjects also received a one-page handout that showed an image of correct probe placement on the body as well as an ideal ultrasound image for each of the three components of the ACT exam. No additional instruction on the ultrasound exam, including probe orientation, anatomy, image quality, or image interpretation, was performed as the study examined the ability to guide a true novice. After the tutorial, the subject ultrasonographer donned the GG, and a connection was established with the expert sonographer stationed in another room. FaceTime connection was also established; however, this device was positioned to show only the ultrasound screen at all times. The expert anesthesiologist visualized both the FT and GG streams on a notebook computer (MacBook Pro 2013). Goggle Glass provided a one-way video and two-way audio communication. FaceTime provided two-way audio and video communication. The expert instructed the ultrasonographer via the GG device.

A SonoSite (Bothell, WA) Edge I system with a 12 MHz linear transducer and a 2–5 MHz phased-array transducer was used for all ultrasound exams. All exams were performed on the same human model, who was a young, healthy male with normal body habitus. A research assistant was present to support any technical issues with communication devices or the ultrasound equipment. Each subject had up to 5 min to complete each of the three ultrasound exams. A five-point scale, as described previously [24], was used, with the value of 3 representing the cut-off score for images deemed suitable for interpretation. The remote expert examiner would stop the subject after an ideal image was achieved (based on the remote examiner's judgment for having an image score ≥3) or if the 5 min exam period elapsed. The expert examiner would score the live image quality for each of three exams immediately after image acquisition.

Additionally, the audio and video feed on the expert examiner's computer was recorded for offline review by a blinded second expert examiner. Prior to study initiation, the blinded second examiner and the expert study sonographer reviewed five complete ACT exam clips to validate inter-rater scoring reliability. Additionally, the blinded reviewer reviewed the clips of the expert sonographer performing an in-person exam on the model used for this study, taking them as the benchmark for the highest-quality image (5/5). No participants were compensated in any way.

2.5. Primary Outcome Measure

For each of the three components of the ACT exam, the frequency of obtaining an adequate image quality, defined as having a value of 3 or higher, was measured. The goal was to identify adequate image quality for at least 80% of the exams.

2.6. Secondary Outcome Measures

All components of the exams were recorded and compared to the exam time of the expert sonographer's in-person examination. All subjects completed surveys on the ease of use of the telecommunication system and the teleultrasound process. The model also completed surveys regarding the level of comfort during the examination for all examiners. The experience surveys of the model were compared between the subjects and the expert sonographer.

2.7. Sample Size and Statistics

Estimation of sample size was based on a priori assumption of a 40% image acquisition rate of clinically interpretable images (>3/5) of the nonmedical participants without teleultrasound assistance. A sample size of 20 subjects was calculated to increase the image acquisition rate to the target of 80%, assuming a power of 0.80 and alpha 0.05. Descriptive statistics were used to report the image acquisition rate for each of the three components of the ACT exam.

3. Results

A total of 21 nonmedically trained undergraduate students without prior ultrasound experience were recruited and completed the study. The average time to complete the specific exams was as follows: cardiac exam, mean = 4.7 (standard deviation (SD) = 3.6 min); pulmonary exam, mean = 1.6 (SD = 1.2 min); abdominal exam, mean = 2.1 (SD = 1.6 min). The average total time for the exam was 8.5 min (SD = 4.6). A comparison between the live expert examiner and the blinded postexam reviewer showed a 100% agreement between image interpretations. A review of the exams rated as three or greater demonstrated that 87% of abdominal, 90% of cardiac, and 95% of pulmonary exams achieved this level of image quality (Figure 2). The complete distribution of the image quality results for each exam type is shown in Figure 3. Standardized patient comfort survey results showed 5/5 scores for all ultrasound examinations. Summary data from the satisfaction survey of the teleultrasound communication by the novice users was as follows on a 5-point Likert scale: audio quality, median = 3.0 (interquartile range (IQR) = 2); ease of following commands, median = 5 (IQR = 1); comfort in obtaining cardiac view, median = 5 (IQR = 1); comfort in obtaining lung view, median = 5 (IQR = 1); and comfort in obtaining abdominal view, median = 4 (IQR = 1).

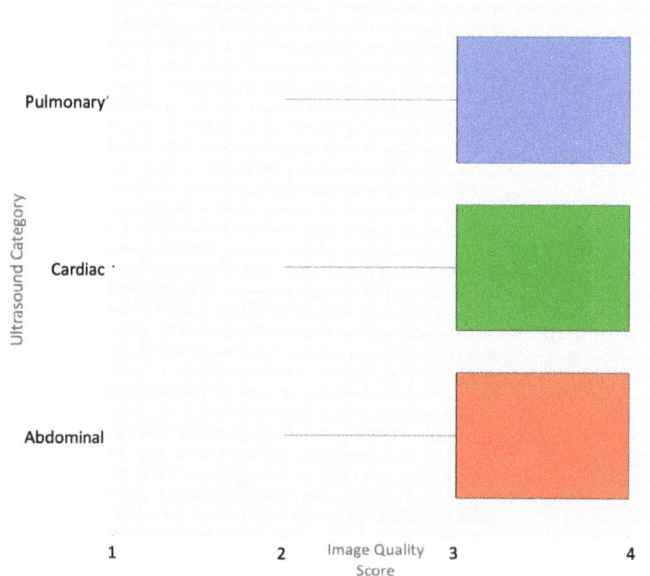

Figure 2. Box plot of image quality scores by ultrasound category.

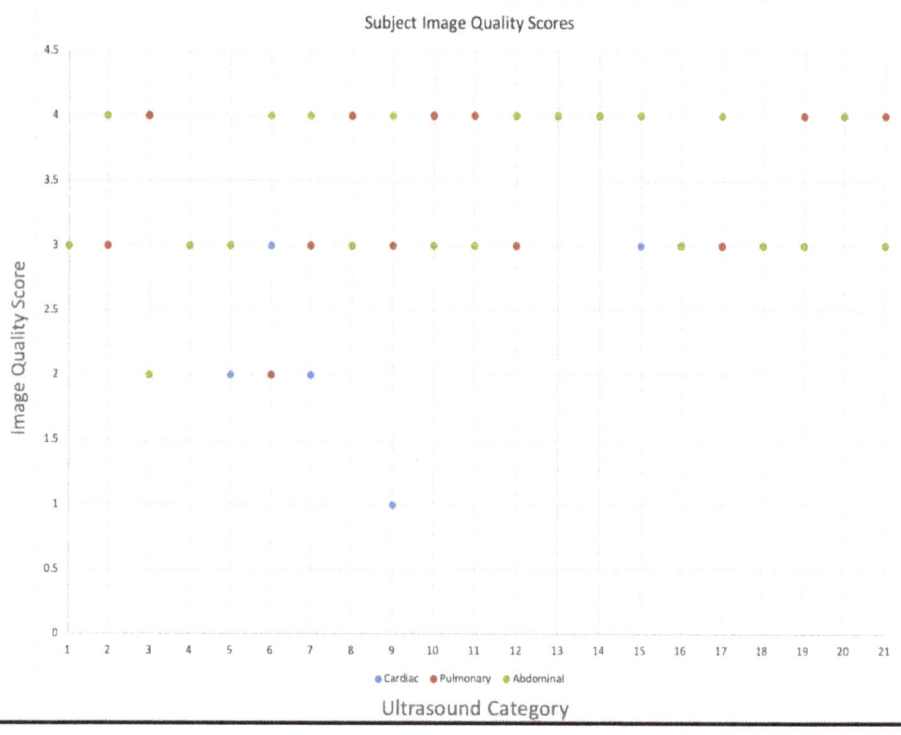

Figure 3. Complete subject image quality scores.

4. Discussion

This pilot study suggests that nonmedical individuals can be directed to complete an acute care POCUS exam using the combination of a POV hands-free audio-visual device (GG) with a commercially available smartphone video conferencing platform (FT). As the technology and cost of medical ultrasound continue to improve, the expansion of its role in healthcare needs to be explored. By combining POCUS technologies with commercially available video communication technologies, one can evaluate new areas to implement portable ultrasound.

Multiple studies have demonstrated the ability to use teleultrasound to connect healthcare providers across vast distances and between rural areas and those in larger medical centers [25]. For example, the ability to instruct paramedics to perform a trauma POCUS examination via real-time physician guidance has been demonstrated [26]. Additionally, Sheehan et al. demonstrated the ability to remotely guide inexperienced users through an ultrasound examination with the application of a visual guidance system [27]. Indeed, the ability to perform POCUS exams in space via remote guidance has also been proven [28]. Further efforts have continued to demonstrate that teleultrasound allows end-users to perform ultrasound examinations with minimal training [25] and that these examinations generate clinically useful ultrasound images for a variety of organ systems and pathologies [25].

As teleultrasound continues to grow, exploration of how this concept can be applied using low-cost, commercially available products have recently been explored. Multiple studies have demonstrated the utility of smartphone-based video conferencing platforms to remotely instruct POCUS examinations [10,16,29]. Images obtained from these platforms are noninferior to those obtained directly from the ultrasound device [18]. In addition, wearable video conferencing devices, such as GG, have also been applied to POCUS applications. For example, the utility of GG for assistance with central venous access has been demonstrated [30].

However, few studies have examined the combination of a wearable video conferencing device (GG) and a smartphone video conferencing platform (FT) to remotely guide nonmedical participants to perform an acute care POCUS examination. This combination is novel and provides a hands-free strategy to provide remote guidance. Additionally, this study demonstrates a cost-effective teleultrasound system that can provide successful remote guidance as well as real-time remote image interpretation. Moreover, our data supports that the time to perform these examinations is practical for acute care management. Indeed, with the rapid cost reduction in teleultrasound technologies and the data demonstrated in our study, further research should explore ways to apply POCUS in new patient care settings. For instance, many public health and international medical mission trips include personnel without medical training. Teleultrasound may increase the contribution of these individuals.

Additionally, this study is also one of the first demonstrating the ability of a perioperative physician to facilitate the use of ultrasound technology outside of the hospital setting. Within the limits of this small, simulation-based study, our results suggest that an appropriately trained anesthesiologist can effectively provide guidance via the described teleultrasound system. This is relevant given the continuous pressure on the specialty of anesthesiology to expand its role in the patient care continuum.

While this study did not assess the application of this system toward patient care, our positive results support the need for additional studies in this area. Specifically, how these low-cost technologies can be used to improve the quality of care in resource-limited environments should be evaluated.

This study has several limitations. It is a small pilot project designed to evaluate the feasibility of a POCUS-trained anesthesiologist to use commercially available teleultrasound technologies. Future studies should evaluate this utility over a larger sample size that is applied over a region more common to traditional telemedicine platforms. In addition, all studies were performed on the same model (both by the expert and participants) to remove the confounding variable of different acoustic windows in patients. No evaluation of pathology was assessed in the study; rather, the focus was on the ability to generate an image that was interpretable remotely with the described teleultrasound technology. Finally, the participants were not tested on the anatomy or interpretation of the image.

5. Conclusions

This pilot project demonstrated the utility of a novel teleultrasound system to guide nonmedically trained adults to successfully acquire ultrasound images useful for acute cardiac, pulmonary, and abdominal assessments. This novel system utilizes low-cost, commercially available technologies and allows the examiner to communicate hands-free. Further studies should evaluate how this described system can be utilized to expand the role of teleultrasound.

Author Contributions: Conceptualization, D.R., M.M., D.Q.L., W.D., and C.R.; methodology, D.R., M.M., D.Q.L., W.D., C.R., M.R., and B.A.; formal analysis, D.R., B.A., and M.R.; software, D.Q.L., M.R., and B.A.; investigation, D.R., M.M., D.Q.L., W.D., and C.R.; writing, D.R., M.M., D.Q.L., W.D., C.R., M.R., and B.A.; project administration, D.R., M.M., C.R., M.R., and B.A.

Funding: This research received no external funding.

Conflicts of Interest: D.R. is a consultant for Fujifilm SonoSite and a member of the Medical Advisory Board of EchoNous. He is also a consultant for General Electric and is carrying out research funded by the company.

References

1. Kumar, R.K. Technology and healthcare costs. *Ann. Pediatr. Cardiol.* **2011**, *4*, 84–86. [CrossRef]
2. Alpert, J.S.; Mladenovic, J.; Hellmann, D.B. Should a hand-carried ultrasound machine become standard equipment for every internist? *Am. J. Med.* **2009**, *122*, 1–3. [CrossRef] [PubMed]
3. Prescient & Strategic Intelligence. Point-of-Care Ultrasound (Pocus) Device Market to Grow at 6.9% Cagr Till 2025: P&s Market Research. Available online: Https://globenewswire.Com/news-release/2017/07/21/1055557/0/en/point-of-care-ultrasound-pocus-device-market-to-grow-at-6-9-cagr-till-2025-p-s-market-research.Html (accessed on 25 September 2019).
4. Moore, C.; Copel, J. Point-of-care ultrasonography. *N. Engl. J. Med.* **2011**, *364*, 749–757. [CrossRef] [PubMed]
5. Kendall, J.L.; Hoffenberg, S.R.; Smith, R.S. History of emergency and critical care ultrasound: The evolution of a new imaging paradigm. *Crit. Care Med.* **2007**, *35*, S126–S130. [CrossRef] [PubMed]
6. Arntfield, R.T.; Millington, S.J. Point of care cardiac ultrasound applications in the emergency department and intensive care unit—A review. *Curr. Cardiol. Rev.* **2012**, *8*, 98–108. [CrossRef] [PubMed]
7. Manno, E.; Navarra, M.; Faccio, L.; Motevallian, M.; Bertolaccini, L.; Mfochive, A.; Pesce, M.; Evangelista, A. Deep impact of ultrasound in the intensive care unit: The "icu-sound" protocol. *Anesthesiology* **2012**, *117*, 801–809. [CrossRef] [PubMed]
8. Ramsingh, D.; Rinehart, J.; Kain, Z.; Strom, S.; Canales, C.; Alexander, B.; Capatina, A.; Ma, M.; Le, K.V.; Cannesson, M. Impact assessment of perioperative point-of-care ultrasound training on anesthesiology residents. *Anesthesiology* **2015**, *123*, 670–682. [CrossRef] [PubMed]
9. Levine, A.R.; McCurdy, M.T.; Zubrow, M.T.; Papali, A.; Mallemat, H.A.; Verceles, A.C. Tele-intensivists can instruct non-physicians to acquire high-quality ultrasound images. *J. Crit. Care* **2015**, *30*, 871–875. [CrossRef]
10. Robertson, T.E.; Levine, A.R.; Verceles, A.C.; Buchner, J.A.; Lantry, J.H., 3rd; Papali, A.; Zubrow, M.T.; Colas, L.N.; Augustin, M.E.; McCurdy, M.T.; et al. Remote tele-mentored ultrasound for non-physician learners using facetime: A feasibility study in a low-income country. *J. Crit. Care* **2017**, *40*, 145–148. [CrossRef]
11. Armstrong, D.G.; Giovinco, N.; Mills, J.L.; Rogers, L.C. Facetime for physicians: Using real time mobile phone-based videoconferencing to augment diagnosis and care in telemedicine. *Eplasty* **2011**, *11*, e23.
12. Chang, J.Y.; Tsui, L.Y.; Yeung, K.S.; Yip, S.W.; Leung, G.K. Surgical vision: Google glass and surgery. *Surg. Innov.* **2016**, *23*, 422–426. [CrossRef] [PubMed]
13. Robinson, M.D.; Branham, A.R.; Locklear, A.; Robertson, S.; Gridley, T. Measuring satisfaction and usability of facetime for virtual visits in patients with uncontrolled diabetes. *Telemed. J. E-Health* **2016**, *22*, 138–143. [CrossRef] [PubMed]
14. Wu, X.; Oliveria, S.A.; Yagerman, S.; Chen, L.; DeFazio, J.; Braun, R.; Marghoob, A.A. Feasibility and efficacy of patient-initiated mobile teledermoscopy for short-term monitoring of clinically atypical nevi. *JAMA Derm.* **2015**, *151*, 489–496. [CrossRef] [PubMed]
15. Williams, G.W.; Buendia, F.I.; Idowu, O.O. Utilization of a mobile videoconferencing tool (facetime) for real-time evaluation of critically ill neurosurgical patients. *J. Neurosurg. Anesthesiol.* **2015**, *27*, 72. [CrossRef] [PubMed]

16. Miyashita, T.; Iketani, Y.; Nagamine, Y.; Goto, T. Facetime((r)) for teaching ultrasound-guided anesthetic procedures in remote place. *J. Clin. Monit. Comput.* **2014**, *28*, 211–215. [CrossRef]
17. Van Oeveren, L.; Donner, J.; Fantegrossi, A.; Mohr, N.M.; Brown, C.A., 3rd. Telemedicine-assisted intubation in rural emergency departments: A national emergency airway registry study. *Telemed. J. E-Health* **2017**, *23*, 290–297. [CrossRef]
18. Levine, A.R.; Buchner, J.A.; Verceles, A.C.; Zubrow, M.T.; Mallemat, H.A.; Papali, A.; McCurdy, M.T. Ultrasound images transmitted via facetime are non-inferior to images on the ultrasound machine. *J. Crit. Care* **2016**, *33*, 51–55. [CrossRef]
19. Zennaro, F.; Neri, E.; Nappi, F.; Grosso, D.; Triunfo, R.; Cabras, F.; Frexia, F.; Norbedo, S.; Guastalla, P.; Gregori, M.; et al. Real-time tele-mentored low cost "point-of-care us" in the hands of paediatricians in the emergency department: Diagnostic accuracy compared to expert radiologists. *PLoS ONE* **2016**, *11*, e0164539. [CrossRef]
20. Kim, C.; Kang, B.S.; Choi, H.J.; Lim, T.H.; Oh, J.; Chee, Y. Clinical application of real-time tele-ultrasonography in diagnosing pediatric acute appendicitis in the ed. *Am. J. Emerg. Med.* **2015**, *33*, 1354–1359. [CrossRef]
21. Anton, D.; Kurillo, G.; Yang, A.Y.; Bajcsy, R. Augmented Telemedicine Platform for Real-Time Remote Medical Consultation. In Proceedings of the 23rd International Conference (MMM), Reykjavík, Iceland, 4–6 January 2017; pp. 77–89.
22. Avgousti, S.; Panayides, A.S.; Christoforou, E.G.; Argyrou, A.; Jossif, A.; Masouras, P.; Vieyres, P. Medical telerobotics and the remote ultrasonography paradigm over 4g wireless networks. In Proceedings of the 2018 IEEE 20th International Conference on e-Health Networking, Applications and Services (Healthcom), Ostrava, Czech, 17–20 September 2018; pp. 1–6.
23. Ramsingh, D.; Alexander, B.; Le, K.; Williams, W.; Canales, C.; Cannesson, M. Comparison of the didactic lecture with the simulation/model approach for the teaching of a novel perioperative ultrasound curriculum to anesthesiology residents. *J. Clin. Anesth.* **2014**, *26*, 443–454. [CrossRef]
24. Jakobsen, C.J.; Torp, P.; Sloth, E. Perioperative feasibility of imaging the heart and pleura in patients with aortic stenosis undergoing aortic valve replacement. *Eur. J. Anaesthesiol.* **2007**, *24*, 589–595. [CrossRef] [PubMed]
25. Britton, N.; Miller, M.A.; Safadi, S.; Siegel, A.; Levine, A.R.; McCurdy, M.T. Tele-ultrasound in resource-limited settings: A systematic review. *Front. Public Health* **2019**, *7*, 244. [CrossRef] [PubMed]
26. Boniface, K.S.; Shokoohi, H.; Smith, E.R.; Scantlebury, K. Tele-ultrasound and paramedics: Real-time remote physician guidance of the focused assessment with sonography for trauma examination. *Am. J. Emerg. Med.* **2011**, *29*, 477–481. [CrossRef] [PubMed]
27. Sheehan, F.H.; Ricci, M.A.; Murtagh, C.; Clark, H.; Bolson, E.L. Expert visual guidance of ultrasound for telemedicine. *J. Telemed. Telecare* **2010**, *16*, 77–82. [CrossRef]
28. Sargsyan, A.E.; Hamilton, D.R.; Jones, J.A.; Melton, S.; Whitson, P.A.; Kirkpatrick, A.W.; Martin, D.; Dulchavsky, S.A. Fast at mach 20: Clinical ultrasound aboard the international space station. *J. Trauma Acute Care Surg.* **2005**, *58*, 35–39. [CrossRef]
29. Smith, A.; Addison, R.; Rogers, P.; Stone-McLean, J.; Boyd, S.; Hoover, K.; Pollard, M.; Dubrowski, A.; Parsons, M. Remote mentoring of point-of-care ultrasound skills to inexperienced operators using multiple telemedicine platforms: Is a cell phone good enough? *J. Ultrasound Med.* **2018**, *37*, 2517–2525. [CrossRef]
30. Wu, T.S.; Dameff, C.J.; Tully, J.L. Ultrasound-guided central venous access using google glass. *J. Emerg. Med.* **2014**, *47*, 668–675. [CrossRef]

© 2019 by the authors. Licensee MDPI, Basel, Switzerland. This article is an open access article distributed under the terms and conditions of the Creative Commons Attribution (CC BY) license (http://creativecommons.org/licenses/by/4.0/).

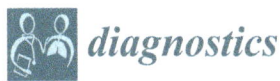

Article

Stakeholders' Perspectives for the Development of a Point-of-Care Diagnostics Curriculum in Rural Primary Clinics in South Africa—Nominal Group Technique

Nkosinothando Chamane [1,*], Desmond Kuupiel [1] and Tivani Phosa Mashamba-Thompson [1,2]

1. Department of Public Health Medicine, School of Nursing and Public Health, University of KwaZulu-Natal, Durban 4041, South Africa; desmondkuupiel98@hotmail.com (D.K.); Mashamba-Thompson@ukzn.ac.za (T.P.M.-T.)
2. Department of Public Health, University of Limpopo, Polokwane 0723, South Africa
* Correspondence: thandocharmane@yahoo.com; Tel.: +27-0760133775

Received: 6 December 2019; Accepted: 7 January 2020; Published: 1 April 2020

Abstract: Poor knowledge and adherence to point-of-care (POC) HIV testing standards have been reported in rural KwaZulu-Natal (KZN), a high HIV prevalent setting. Improving compliance to HIV testing standards is critical, particularly during the gradual phasing out of lay counsellor providers and the shifting of HIV testing and counselling duties to professional nurses. The main objective of this study was to identify priority areas for development of POC diagnostics curriculum to improve competence and adherence to POC diagnostics quality standards for primary healthcare (PHC) nurses in rural South Africa. Method: PHC clinic stakeholders were invited to participate in a co-creation workshop. Participants were purposely sampled from each of the 11 KwaZulu-Natal Districts. Through the Nominal Group Technique (NGT), participants identified training related challenges concerning delivery of quality point of care diagnostics and ranked them from highest to lowest priority. An importance ranking score (scale 1–5) was calculated for each of the identified challenges. Results: Study participants included three PHC professional nurses, one TB professional nurse, one HIV lay councilor, one TB assistant and three POC diagnostics researchers, aged 23–50. Participants identified ten POC diagnostics related challenges. Amongst the highest ranked challenges were the following:absence of POC testing Curriculum for nurses, absence of training of staff on HIV testing and counselling as lay counsellor providers are gradually being phased out,. absence of Continuous Professional Development opportunities and lack of Staff involvement in POC Management programs. Conclusion: Key stakeholders perceived training of PHC nurses as the highest priority for the delivery of quality POC diagnostic testing at PHC level. We recommend continual collaboration among all POC diagnostics stakeholders in the development of an accessible curriculum to improve providers' competence and ensure sustainable quality delivery of POC diagnostic services in rural PHC clinics.

Keywords: quality HIV point-of-care-diagnostics; nominal group technique; stakeholder engagement

1. Introduction

Point-of-care (POC) diagnostic testing is defined as timely clinical testing performed during patient consultation when the result will be used to take appropriate action, which will lead to an improved health outcome [1]. POC diagnostic testing plays a critical role in healthcare access in settings with limited laboratory infrastructure. Early diagnosis and rapid initiation of treatment is key to controlling infectious diseases including HIV/AIDS [1,2]. Improving the quality of diagnostic services is therefore essential for improved access to quality primary healthcare (PHC) services. In South Africa an HIV Counselling and Testing (HCT) campaign was first launched in April 2010. During this time in

PHC clinics HIV/AIDS testing was done by lay counselors, who were permanently employed staff sent for training specific to performing HIV/AIDS rapid testing and counselling. Their role was solely to provide HIV testing and counselling services. In 2014 the South African Department of Health then announced the gradual phasing out of lay councilors and adding HIV testing duties to professional nurse consultation duties. This shift of duties may lead to added pressure on clinics who already suffer because of staff shortages. Moreover, poor knowledge and adherence to quality assurance as well as HIV testing standards remain a challenge especially in resource limited areas [3]. This is a concern because quality assurance programs, which include regular calibration of instruments, participation to external quality assessment schemes, adherence to standard operating procedures and test operator competency as well as running of internal quality control samples on every test day have been shown to ensure accuracy of POC diagnostic testing [4,5]. Factors contributing to this problem include poor access to laboratory infrastructure, training resources and institutions due to clinics being situated in deep rural areas, time constraints and lack of motivation to engage in new interventions [3,6,7].

Various initiatives have been introduced towards addressing this challenge. They include the Rapid HIV testing quality improvement initiative (RTQII) introduced to seven countries in 2013, including Tanzania, Ethiopia and Kenya [8]. The goal of RTQII was to scale up coverage of HIV rapid testing quality improvement (QI) and assurance activities as well as to improve the quality and safety of rapid testing services [8]. The RTQII findings emphasized provision of standard operating procedures (SOPs), onsite supervision, job aiders and orientation of providers on the importance of compliance to HIV rapid testing standards as the main tactics which led to quality improvement [9].

In this study, we involved PHC clinic-based POC diagnostics stakeholders in a co-creation workshop to identify priority areas for the development of point-of-care (POC) diagnostics curriculum to improve competence and adherence to POC diagnostics quality standards for PHC nurses in rural South Africa. The findings of this study have the potential to inform policy making concerning Continuous Professional Development (CPD) interventions aimed at improving the competency of PHC health workers on POC diagnostics services. This will further contribute towards healthcare systems strengthening, through improving and ensuring provision of quality, reliable and sustainable POC diagnostic services.

2. Materials and Methods

2.1. Study Design

The Nominal Group Technique (NGT) was employed to enable engagement with representative key stakeholders from 11 districts of KwaZulu Natal (KZN). We defined key stakeholders as PHC workers with experience in performing POC diagnostic services in rural KZN PHC clinics and researchers in the field of POC diagnostics. NGT is defined as a process to identify strategic problems and to develop appropriate and innovative interventions to address them [10]. The NGT processes is commonly applied to homogenous groups and it involves four main phases—(i) Nominal or silent phase, where participants individually consider their personal responses to a presented question and write them down; (ii) Item generation phase, where individual participants take turns to share their responses with the group. The items generated are recorded without being discussed; (iii) Discussion and clarification phase, where group members discuss and ask questions in order to clarify items on the list and elaborate on their responses. During this phase, items with similar meanings are combined and duplicate items can be removed; (iv) Voting phase, here each participant is asked to prioritize the listed items by assigning ranks to them. The ranking results are then collated to produce a single list of priorities for the wider group [11,12]. Application of this process in this study is discussed below.

2.1.1. Study Participants

We invited key stakeholders of PHC-based POC diagnostics to participate in a Nominal group co-creation workshop. The NGT team comprised of three Professional nurses, one TB professional nurse, one TB assistant, one HIV/AIDS lay councilor, two experienced researchers, the primary researcher (as facilitator) and one research assistant. Detailed characteristics of participants are presented in the next section.

2.1.2. Sampling Strategy

A purposeful sampling strategy was used to select representative clinics to participate in this study. This sampling technique involves identifying and selecting participants with practical knowledge and experience of PHC-based POC diagnostics. This study was conducted as a follow up to the cross-sectional survey of 100 randomly selected clinics in KZN rural PHC clinics [3,13]. The survey was aimed at demining the accessibility, availability and utility of POC diagnostic services in rural PHC clinics [13]. Clinics identified to have the highest availability and usage of POC diagnostics following the survey were selected to participate in this study. We thus included one PHC clinic from each of the 11 KZN districts with the highest availability and usage of POC tests. Clinics with low HIV POC diagnostics availability and usage were excluded due to minimal experience in HIV testing as reported in a previous audit [3].

2.1.3. NGT Process

The PI (NC) facilitated the workshop with the help of a trained research assistant (PS). The four phase NGT was performed to achieve the objective of this study. Prior to the meeting of all key stakeholders, a pre-elicitation technique [14] was employed, where collaborators were sent an invitation together with a brief on the program of the day. The brief included the purpose to create a platform for key stakeholders to come together and determine training-related challenges affecting delivery of quality point of care diagnostics services in PHC clinics and to identify priority areas to be addressed in order to overcome the challenges. The main aim of the NGT was to bring together key stakeholders to identify priority areas for the development of a POC diagnostics curriculum.

At the opening of the session all participants were given an opportunity to introduce themselves, sharing their current positions as well as the number of years of experience in the field of HIV/AIDS testing. Following this, the PI (NC) provided a background to the workshop and presented the program of the day as illustrated in Figure 1. The participants were then separated into two sub-groups of four. The sub-groups were provided with a set of sticky notes, pens, markers and a flip chart sheet.

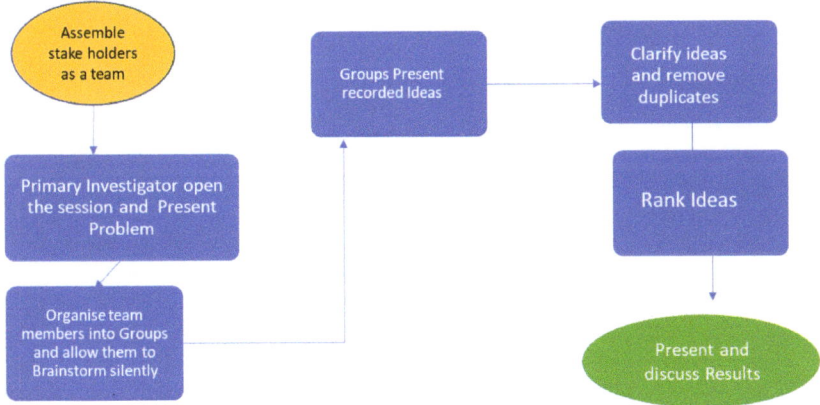

Figure 1. Nominal Group Technique (NGT) session to identify training related challenges with the delivery of quality point of care diagnostics.

The PI (NC) posed the following question to participants, to start the workshop: what training related challenges do you encounter with regards to the delivery of quality HIV/AIDS Rapid tests? The following steps were followed to answer this question:

2.1.4. Silent Brainstorming

Participants were given up to 10 min to consider the question and note down all the relevant ideas that came to mind. Discussions were prohibited during this period, however the participants could raise their hands for the attention of the facilitator if in need of clarity on the above question.

2.1.5. Group Discussion

Group members were given another 10 min to share their ideas within their groups, group them into themes as they emerged and then stick them on the flip chart sheet to be presented to the whole workshop group.

2.1.6. Group Presentations and Clarification

Each sub-group selected one representative to present their ideas according to the themes they had agreed upon. The facilitator encouraged questions and discussions during the discussion sessions. This process was also used as an opportunity to probe the presenters for further explanations as well as for the wider team to discuss and clarify presented ideas. During this process the research assistant collated all the ideas and together with the facilitator highlighted similar themes and removed duplicates. The collated results were presented to the wider group as priority areas to be ranked during the ranking session.

2.1.7. Ranking of Ideas

The ranking process followed the strategy suggested by Delbecq et al. [15] of ranking ideas through assigning a value to an idea according to its priority. Ranking is usually preferred by many researchers, because scores can be quickly tallied and the results can be interpreted and discussed within the same session [16]. Participants were given a break, while the facilitator through the use of an online form software (Google® Forms, Google LLC, Mountain View, CA, USA) with the help of a trained research assistant created a ranking questionnaire. The questionnaire consisted of 11 challenges presented by the two groups combined.

The questionnaire was handed to each participant for ranking ideas using a Likert scale of 1–5 scores with 1 representing very low priority and 5 representing highest priority. The ranking process was conducted independently and without discussion. The results were collated and analyzed using a spreadsheet as explained in the data analysis section below.

2.1.8. Data Management

During the nominal group discussions, two types of data were collected; qualitative and quantitative data. Each type of data obtained was first managed individually and then the findings were combined to fully address the main aim of this study. Qualitative data was recorded in chart sheets as well as through a recorder to be analyzed at a later stage. Quantitative data obtained from the ranking tool was entered onto a google spreadsheet for further analysis as explained in the section below. This enabled us to immediately report the results back to the participants and more qualitative data was obtained during clarification to elaborate on the ranking data

2.2. Data Analysis

Two nominal groups consisting of four participants each were conducted. Data analysis was ongoing and an overview of the process followed is provided in Figure 2. This involved ranking of ideas and thematic analysis of the qualitative data. All stages are described in detail below, where analysis will be discussed in the context of three terms: ideas, priorities and themes [12].

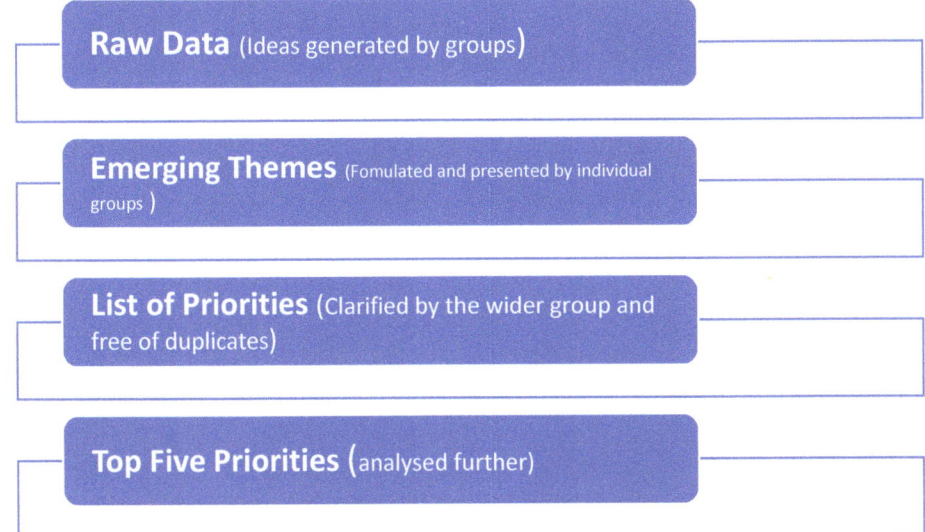

Figure 2. Overview of the NGT Data analysis Process.

2.2.1. Raw Data Analysis

Ideas raised by participants in the silent brainstorming of each nominal group were presented to the wider group. All the ideas were put up for participants to view simultaneously and the facilitator went on to facilitate grouping of all the ideas according to emerging themes agreed upon by the wider group. Similar ideas were grouped together and duplicates were removed. The themes then became priorities to be voted upon in the ranking stage.

2.2.2. Quantitative Data Analysis

The most common technique to analyze and describe nominal group data is summing the votes allocated to each idea to determine the overall priority score [17–19]. This method was employed in this study, where quantitative data obtained from the participants ranking of ideas on a scale of 1–5 was analyzed through the summing of votes allocated to each idea. The overall priority score for each theme was then calculated. This was done through capturing ranking responses into google forms and calculating overall priority scores. A priority list of responses was then drawn and presented to the wider group.

2.2.3. Qualitative Data Analysis

We conducted qualitative analysis of the first five highest overall priority scores. The recorded qualitative data were collected from the participant's presentations, where the rationale for selecting these themes was provided. More qualitative data collected during the discussion and clarification of the priority list was also utilized to elaborate more on the selected themes.

3. Results

3.1. Characteristics of Study Participants

In total the NGT team comprised of 8 participants from ages 23–50, with each group comprising of four participants. The attendance rate was 72% since 11 participants were expected. Reasons for nonattendance included other work commitments, inability to organise transportation, other appointments and protest actions on the road. All the stakeholders in attendance reported involvement in POC diagnostics and their specific roles are reported in Table 1.

Table 1. Key stakeholder characteristics and involvement in point-of-care (POC) diagnostic services.

District/Institution	Occupation	POC Diagnostics Involvement
Umgungundlovu	Professional Nurse	Testing and HIV Program co-Ordinator
Harry Gwala	Professional Nurse	Full patient consultations, including HIV testing
Uthukela	Professional Nurse	Full patient consultations, including HIV testing
Umzinyathi	TB Professional Nurse	TB and HIV testing
Ilembe	HIV/AIDS lay councillor	HIV Testing
Ethekwini	TB assistant	Previous HIV lay counsellor
University of KZN	Academic Leader	Medical Scientist, Public Health Professor with expertise on implementation research for POC diagnostics
University of KZN	Postdoctoral Fellow	Researcher in implementation and supply chain management of POC diagnostic tests

3.2. Nominal Group Ranking

Stakeholders identified a combined total of 18 challenges (Appendix A), which were then categorised into 10 themes. Ranking results of these themes from highest priority to lowest are presented in Table 2.

Table 2. Ranking results in descending order.

Item	Summing by Votes Scores					Total%
	5	4	3	2	1	100
No POC Testing Curriculum for nurses	7	2	0	1	0	90
No training of staff on HIV testing and counselling as lay counsellors are being phased out.	7	0	2	1	0	86
Continuous Professional Development	6	1	3	0	0	84
HPIC Tracking and registering patients before testing: Correct Record Keeping	6	2	0	1	1	82
Staff involvement in POC Management program	5	2	2	0	1	80
Pressure on lay councillors due to staff shortage and having to meet targets	4	3	1	1	1	76
Supply Chain Management for POC diagnostics testing	4	3	1	1	1	76
Confidentiality-Stigma	4	2	2	1	1	74
Research Study Process control: Better informed participants to ensure adherence to study timelines	2	1	5	1	1	64
Client Attitude to testing	2	1	5	1	1	64

3.3. Thematic Analysis of Top Five Priorities

The study was aimed at determining priority areas for development of a POC diagnostics curriculum for PHC nurses in rural South Africa. From the ten priority areas determined by key stakeholders during the workshop, the top five ranked priorities were: Absence of POC testing curriculum for nurses (90%); absence of training of staff on HIV testing and counselling as lay counsellors are being phased out (86%); absence of Continuous Professional Development (84%); HPIC Tracking and registering patients before testing: Correct Record Keeping (82%) and Staff involvement in POC Management program (80%). Each theme is presented below with supporting quotes.

3.3.1. Absence of POC Testing Curriculum for Nurses

Stakeholders ranked the absence of a curriculum specific to POC diagnostic services for PHC nurses as the highest challenge to be addressed urgently. The main reasons they highlighted were that personnel who performed HIV testing relied on the knowledge they obtained in their past training, each other's experiences as well as the internet accessed through personal phones. Furthermore, they reported that there were no structured follow-ups to validate what they were doing. Priority is more on getting tests done and meeting targets. When asked about standard operating procedures they responded that these were not available in their clinics and one participant who worked at a clinic that did have one said that SOPs were not readily available and not easily accessible: "not having a standard training is very unfair because we do not even have internet to search when we do not understand something."

3.3.2. Absence of Training of Staff on HIV Testing and Counselling as Lay Counsellors Are Being Phased Out

Stakeholders reported that they were concerned that no formal training was provided to professional nurses in order to gain skills needed for the provision of quality POC testing, particularly during this period of phasing out of lay counsellors. Participants highlighted that lay councillors were well trained to provide high quality HIV testing and counselling services. In addition, the main duty for lay counsellors was HIV testing, therefore all their attention was on providing this service to the best of their ability: "there is a great need to motivate, encourage and re-train Professional nurses to take over the quality duties of phased out HIV/AIDS lay-councillors, because lay councillors provided more quality testing than professional nurses who have other priorities."

3.3.3. Absence of Continuous Professional Development

In addition to not having a POC curriculum, stakeholders reported lack of financial support to enrol on additional courses. Stakeholders reported that the shortage of staff in clinics prevented them from securing leave days to attend workshops. They also reported a lack of such opportunities and that they rarely receive invitations to attend workshops. As a result, PHC professionals rely on secondary information from senior nurses who are usually invited to attend workshops: "majority of Professional nurses obtained their qualifications many years ago, having them just be given HIV testing duties on top of their current workload without some form of training is not right"

"From time to time nurses need to be updated or retrained as new technologies change all the time"

3.3.4. HPRS Tracking and Registering Patients before Testing: Correct Record Keeping

Health Patient Registration System (HPRS) is a tracking system that works via the Health Patient Registration Number (HPRN) with a purpose to track and keep a unique record for each patient. Stakeholders ranked the utility of this system for correct record keeping amongst high priority challenges because there are shortages of HPRS registers and there are no other means to support this system to ensure that correct information is captured. Moreover, this system is not linked across different health centres in the country, which then largely affects the reliability of HIV statistics reported for South Africa.

3.3.5. Lack of Staff Involvement in POC Management Programs

Stakeholders who were still on their lay-counsellor duties expressed their disappointment by the lack of interest of professional nurses on POC Management programs. Amongst these programs they highlighted procurement, quality assurance and proficiency testing: "professional nurses always complain about how overworked they are as it is, adding HIV testing on top of all that they have to do is really worrying"; "POC management programs will suffer even more with having no one whose main focus is HIV testing"

4. Discussion

This study has identified priority areas for the development of a POC diagnostics curriculum to improve competence and adherence to POC diagnostics quality standards for primary healthcare (PHC) nurses in rural South Africa. From the five highest ranked priorities, four concern the absence of training, Continuing Professional development (CPD) opportunities for PHC professionals and poor staff involvement in HIV programs. The fourth highest ranked priority (HPRS Tracking and registering patients before testing: Correct Record Keeping) is the only priority addressing a different issue. However, this particular priority is a significant and very interesting finding to be looked at further, as it touches issues of record keeping and HIV statistics in the country. The findings of this study also identified gaps in the management and proper implementation of HIV diagnostics in South Africa. This is particularly due to the phasing out of HIV lay counsellors and adding HIV testing to professional nurse duties without a structured training in place to ensure proper transition as well as the sustainability of quality testing services. The findings of this study also demonstrate that identifying of priority areas towards improving the quality of POC diagnostic services has an impact on the achievement of the 90:90:90 goal by 2020, which is a local health priority. In recent years South Africa has made great progress in getting more people tested for HIV; where in 2017 the first of the 90-90-90 targets was met, with 90% of people living with HIV being aware of their status up from 66.2% in 2014 [20,21]. The statistics look impressive, however achieving these targets may lead to increased pressure on nurses performing HIV rapid tests, which could compromise the quality of tests performed as highlighted by the stake holders in this study.

The findings of this study support the wider literature in emphasizing that incompetency of health professionals, lack of CPD, training resources and time constraints remain as barriers to the provision of quality POC services in resource limited settings [3,4,22]. Furthermore, participants in a study conducted in a resource limited setting in India also highlighted high workloads, lack of willingness to participate in POC testing programs, missing support (including training) and pressure to meet targets as contributors to poor quality testing [23]. A report focusing the spotlight on the full achievement of the 90:90:90 goal highlighted healthcare workers attitudes as one of the barriers for patients who want to know their HIV status as well as those who want to return to care [24]. Stakeholder who participated in our study also raised concerns about poor health worker attitudes and lack of staff involvement in HIV management programs as a result of lack of training or too much work pressure, as lay counsellors are being phased out.

In comparison to other research approaches like focus group discussions and in-depth interviews, Stakeholder engagements through the NGT were shown to be effective in identifying priority areas for the development of a POC diagnostics Curriculum. Furthermore, the findings of this study support findings of recent studies conducted in a similar setting [2,3,21,22]. These studies also highlighted lack of support, training opportunities, high workloads and lack of staff involvement as challenges or priority arears to be addressed towards ensuring the provision of quality POC diagnostic services. Stakeholder engagements were further recommended for ensuring effectiveness of future diagnostics as well as for the true potential of POC testing to be realized [4,23].

Strengths of this study include that healthcare users' views and priorities are increasingly being recognized by policy makers in contributing towards improvement of current policies and practices [12]. A limitation to this study in comparison to other NGT studies may be due to poor availability of stakeholders from four KZN districts, however the participating stakeholders represented a wide variety of relevant role players in the implementation of POC diagnostic services. Moreover, since there were only two groups, all the participants had a fair opportunity to express their views and more time was available for probing and clarifying of ideas. Furthermore, there were no challenges in terms of comparing and presenting larger data sets, which is normally the case for multiple group NGTs [12,25].

Recommendations

Based on the success of the NGT in identifying and ranking priority areas with supporting reasons for the development of a POC curriculum for nurses in rural clinics, we recommend more stakeholder involvement in the development of a context specific POC diagnostic services curriculum for onsite training. This curriculum must be supported by the availability of quality assures in each clinic and regular meetings for staff members to review SOPs and discuss POC diagnostics related issues with management to ensure sustainability.

5. Conclusions

This study has presented key stakeholders' views on the development of a POC diagnostics curriculum to improve competence and adherence to POC diagnostics quality standards for primary healthcare (PHC) nurses in rural South Africa. Phasing out of HIV lay counsellors without a POC curriculum in place, continuous professional development and lack of staff involvement in HIV testing programs were ranked as the highest priority areas that need more focus to ensure delivery of quality POC diagnostic testing at the PHC level. We recommend continuous collaborations between all POC diagnostics stakeholders for the development of an effective and accessible curriculum to ensure quality and sustainable POC diagnostic services in rural PHC clinics.

Author Contributions: N.C. and T.P.M.-T. Conceptualized the study. D.K. carried out first data analysis during the NGT. N.C. carried out further data analysis and interpretation of results and then produced the first draft of the manuscript. T.P.M.-T. commented on the draft and contributed to the final version. All authors have read and agreed to the published version of the manuscript.

Funding: This research was funded by University of Kwazulu-Natal College of Health Sciences, grant number 589063.

Acknowledgments: The authors would like to thank all stakeholders, for their time and sharing their knowledge and experiences for the benefit of this study. We would also like to thank the Department of Health KwaZulu-Natal for giving permission for their employees to take time away from their clinical duties to participate in this study as well as the College of Health Sciences, University of KwaZulu-Natal, for resources to assist with setting up and conducting of this research study.

Conflicts of Interest: The authors declare no conflict of interest.

Appendix A

Identified list of Priorities for the development of a POC diagnostics Curriculum

1. Continuous Professional Development
2. POC Testing Curriculum for nurses
3. Staff involvement in POC Management program
4. Understaffing
5. Client Attitude to testing
6. Grand mothering phenomenon
7. Consent for testing children
8. Supply Chain Management for POC diagnostics testing
9. Shortage of equipment
10. Shortage of test kits
11. Research Study Process control: Better informed participants to ensure adherence to study timelines
12. Confidentiality
13. Stigma
14. Pressure on lay councilors due to staff shortage and having to meet targets
15. No training of staff on HIV testing and counselling as lay counsellors are being phased out.
16. HPIC Tracking and registering patients before testing: Correct Record Keeping.
17. Incorrect demographic data
18. Non regular System update

References

1. Pai, N.P.; Vadnais, C.; Denkinger, C.; Engel, N.; Pai, M. Point-of-care testing for infectious diseases: Diversity, complexity and barriers in low-and middle-income countries. *Plos Med.* **2012**, *9*, e1001306. [CrossRef] [PubMed]
2. Smith, M.K.; Rutstein, S.E.; Powers, K.A.; Fidler, S.; Miller, W.C.; Eron, J.J., Jr.; Cohen, M.S. The detection and management of early HIV infection: A clinical and public health emergency. *J. Acquir. Immune Defic. Syndr. (1999)* **2013**, *63*, S187. [CrossRef] [PubMed]

3. Jaya, Z.; Drain, P.K.; Mashamba-Thompson, T.P. Evaluating quality management systems for HIV rapid testing services in primary healthcare clinics in rural KwaZulu-Natal, South Africa. *PLoS ONE* **2017**, *12*, e0183044. [CrossRef] [PubMed]
4. Mashamba-Thompson, T.; Jama, N.; Sartorius, B.; Drain, P.; Thompson, R. Implementation of point-of-care diagnostics in rural primary healthcare clinics in South Africa: Perspectives of key stakeholders. *Diagnostics* **2017**, *7*, 3. [CrossRef] [PubMed]
5. Mashauri, F.; Siza, J.; Temu, M.; Mngara, J.; Kishamawe, C.; Changalucha, J. Assessment of quality assurance in HIV testing in health facilities in Lake Victoria zone, Tanzania. *Tanzan. J. Health Res.* **2007**, *9*, 110–114. [CrossRef] [PubMed]
6. Gray, R.H.; Makumbi, F.; Serwadda, D.; Lutalo, T.; Nalugoda, F.; Opendi, P.; Kigozi, G.; Reynolds, S.J.; Sewankambo, N.K.; Wawer, M.J. Limitations of rapid HIV-1 tests during screening for trials in Uganda: Diagnostic test accuracy study. *Bmj (Clin. Res. Ed.)* **2007**, *335*, 188. [CrossRef] [PubMed]
7. Munyewende, P.O.; Rispel, L.C. Using diaries to explore the work experiences of primary health care nursing managers in two South African provinces. *Glob. Health Action* **2014**, *7*, 1–10. [CrossRef] [PubMed]
8. Nyambo, R.; Hizza, E.; Ntangeki, D. Increasing Accountability for the Reliability of Rapid HIV Test Results: Observations from Seven Facilities in Rungwe District Council, Tanzania. Available online: https://www.usaidassist.org/sites/default/files/assist_tanzania_rtqi_technical_report_mar2018_a4.pdf (accessed on 9 January 2020).
9. FIND. Hiv Rapid Test Quality Improvement Initiative. 2016. Available online: https://www.finddx.org/wp-content/uploads/2016/12/RQTII_project.pdf (accessed on 9 January 2020).
10. Delbecq, A.L.; Van de Ven, A.H. A group process model for problem identification and program planning. *J. Appl. Behav. Sci.* **1971**, *7*, 466–492. [CrossRef]
11. Harvey, N.; Holmes, C.A. Nominal group technique: An effective method for obtaining group consensus. *Int. J. Nurs. Pract.* **2012**, *18*, 188–194. [CrossRef] [PubMed]
12. McMillan, S.S.; Kelly, F.; Sav, A.; Kendall, E.; King, M.A.; Whitty, J.A.; Wheeler, A.J. Using the Nominal Group Technique: How to analyse across multiple groups. *Health Serv. Outcomes Res. Methodol.* **2014**, *14*, 92–108. [CrossRef]
13. Mashamba-Thompson, T.; Sartorius, B.; Drain, P. Operational assessment of point-of-care diagnostics in rural primary healthcare clinics of KwaZulu-Natal, South Africa: A cross-sectional survey. *BMC Health Serv. Res.* **2018**, *18*, 380. [CrossRef] [PubMed]
14. Gonzales, C.K.; Leroy, G. Eliciting user requirements using appreciative inquiry. *Empir. Softw. Eng.* **2011**, *16*, 733–772. [CrossRef]
15. Delbecq, A.L.; Van de Ven, A.H.; Gustafson, D.H. *Group Techniques for Program Planning: A Guide to Nominal Group and Delphi Processes*; Oxford University Press: New York, NY, USA, 1976; p. 338.
16. Poling, R. THE NOMINAL GROUP TECHNIQUE. Available online: https://www.uaex.edu/support-units/program-staff-development/docs/NGTProcess%2012.pdf (accessed on 9 January 2020).
17. Dening, K.H.; Jones, L.; Sampson, E.L. Preferences for end-of-life care: A nominal group study of people with dementia and their family carers. *Palliat. Med.* **2013**, *27*, 409–417. [CrossRef] [PubMed]
18. Hiligsmann, M.; van Durme, C.; Geusens, P.; Dellaert, B.G.; Dirksen, C.D.; van der Weijden, T.; Reginster, J.-Y.; Boonen, A. Nominal group technique to select attributes for discrete choice experiments: An example for drug treatment choice in osteoporosis. *Patient Prefer. Adherence* **2013**, *7*, 133. [CrossRef] [PubMed]
19. Sanderson, T.; Hewlett, S.; Richards, P.; Morris, M.; Calnan, M. Utilizing qualitative data from nominal groups: Exploring the influences on treatment outcome prioritization with rheumatoid arthritis patients. *J. Health Psychol.* **2012**, *17*, 132–142. [CrossRef] [PubMed]
20. Johnson, L.F.; Dorrington, R.E.; Moolla, H. Progress towards the 2020 targets for HIV diagnosis and antiretroviral treatment in South Africa. *S. Afr. J. Hiv Med.* **2017**, *18*. [CrossRef] [PubMed]
21. UNAIDS. UNAIDS DATA 2017. 2017. Available online: https://www.unaids.org/en/resources/documents/2017/2017_data_book (accessed on 9 January 2020).
22. Gaede, B.; Versteeg, M. The state of the right to health in rural South Africa. *South Afr. health Rev.* **2011**, *1*, 99–106.
23. Engel, N.; Ganesh, G.; Patil, M.; Yellappa, V.; Pai, N.P.; Vadnais, C.; Pai, M. Barriers to point-of-care testing in India: Results from qualitative research across different settings, users and major diseases. *PLoS ONE* **2015**, *10*, e0135112. [CrossRef] [PubMed]

24. Gopal, T. In-Depth: The Problem of Stopping or not Starting HIV Treatment. Available online: https://www.google.com.hk/url?sa=t&rct=j&q=&esrc=s&source=web&cd=1&ved=2ahUKEwidp8iSx_XmAhX6wosBHZ_CCP4QFjAAegQIBRAB&url=https%3A%2F%2Fwww.spotlightnsp.co.za%2F2019%2F03%2F06%2Fin-depth-the-problem-of-stopping-or-not-starting-hiv-treatment%2F&usg=AOvVaw3HFvVqkZ9Nv-qvh7zqK5M0 (accessed on 9 January 2020).
25. Sink, D.S. Using the nominal group technique effectively. *Natl. Product. Rev.* **1983**, *2*, 173–184. [CrossRef]

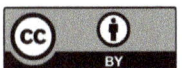

© 2020 by the authors. Licensee MDPI, Basel, Switzerland. This article is an open access article distributed under the terms and conditions of the Creative Commons Attribution (CC BY) license (http://creativecommons.org/licenses/by/4.0/).

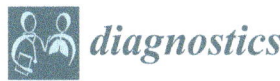

Article

Key Stakeholders' Perspectives on Implementation and Scale up of HIV Self-Testing in Rwanda

Tafadzwa Dzinamarira [1,2,3,*], **Collins Kamanzi** [2] **and Tivani Phosa Mashamba-Thompson** [1,4,5]

1. Department of Public Health Medicine, School of Nursing and Public Health, University of KwaZulu-Natal, Durban 4001, South Africa; Mashamba-Thompson@ukzn.ac.za
2. College of Medicine and Health Sciences, University of Rwanda, Kigali P.O. Box 3286, Rwanda; ckamanzi@nursph.org
3. ICAP, Mailman School of Public Health, Columbia University, Kigali 2807, Rwanda
4. CIHR Canadian HIV Trials Network, Vancouver, BC V6Z 1Y6, Canada
5. Department of Public Health, University of Limpopo, Polokwane, Limpopo 0727, South Africa
* Correspondence: anthonydzina@gmail.com or 219095120@stu.ukzn.ac.za

Received: 20 January 2020; Accepted: 13 February 2020; Published: 1 April 2020

Abstract: Introduction: The World Health Organisation recommends HIV self-testing as an alternative testing method to help reach underserved populations, such as men in sub-Saharan Africa. Successful implementation and scale-up of HIV self-testing (HIVST) in Rwanda relies heavily on relevant stakeholders' involvement. We sought to explore HIVST key stakeholders' perceptions of the implementation and scale-up of HIVST in Rwanda. Method: We conducted in-depth interviews with personnel involved in HIV response projects in Rwanda between September and November 2019. We purposively sampled and interviewed 13 national-level key stakeholders from the Ministry of Health, Rwanda Biomedical Center, non-governmental organizations and HIV clinics at tertiary health facilities in Kigali. We used a thematic approach to analysis with a coding framework guided by Consolidated Framework for Implementation Research (intervention characteristics, inner setting, outer setting, characteristics of individuals involved in the implementation and the implementation process). Results: Key stakeholders perceived HIVST as a potentially effective initiative, which can be used in order to ensure that there is an improvement in uptake of testing services, especially for underserved populations in Rwanda. The following challenges for implementation and scale-up of HIVST were revealed: lack of awareness of the kits, high cost of the self-test kits, and concerns on results interpretation. Key stakeholders identified the following as prerequisites to the successful implementation and scale-up of HIVST in Rwanda; creation of awareness, training those involved in the implementation process, regulation of the selling of the self-test kits, reduction of the costs of acquiring the self-test kits through the provision of subsidies, and ensuring consistent availability of the self-test kits. Conclusions: Key stakeholders expressed confidence in HIVST's ability to improve the uptake of HIV testing services. However, they reported challenges, which need to be addressed to ensure successful implementation and scale-up of the HIVST. There is a need for further research incorporating lower level stakeholders to fully understand HIVST implementation and scale-up challenges and strategies to inform policy.

Keywords: HIV self-testing; implementation; scale-up; key stakeholder

1. Introduction

Globally, it is approximated that only 79% of individuals who live with HIV are aware of their HIV status [1]. In Rwanda, the findings of a 2018–2019 national HIV survey in Rwanda indicated that 17% of adults living with HIV were unaware of their status [2]. By sex; 15% of HIV-positive women and 20% of HIV-positive men did not know their HIV status [2]. Improving the uptake of HIV testing services (HTS) remains one of the main strategies to combating HIV [3,4]. In 2016, the World Health Organization (WHO) provided the first global guidelines on HIV self-testing (HIVST), as an additional model for improving uptake of HTS [5]. Based on statistics from the WHO, 77 nations have adopted HIV self-testing policies, whereas several others are presently developing them [1]. WHO guidelines have been aimed at supporting the implementation and scale-up of ethical, effective, acceptable, as well as evidence-based approaches to HIVST [1]. Along with other sub-Saharan African countries, the Rwanda Ministry of Health in 2017 recommended the use of HIVST as an additional strategy [6].

HIVST refers to the process where an individual collects his own specimen, which could be blood or oral fluid, and thereafter carries out HIV testing and decodes the result, in most cases in a private setting [5]. HIVST has the potential to overcome some of the main barriers which are associated with the current testing models [7–11]. The notable barriers include stigma, discrimination, as well as non-confidential testing environments [7,8]. Acceptability studies have provided mixed findings. In South Africa, a very low rate of acceptability of HIVST (22%) was reported among conveniently-sampled adults [12]. Similarly, low acceptability (44%) was reported in China among men who have sex with men [13]. High acceptability rates have been reported among university students in the Democratic Republic of Congo (82%) [14]; men who have sex with men in Peru and Brazil (87%) [9] and a general adult population in western Kenya (94%) [11]. Globally, it has been documented in various studies that HIVST is acceptable in general populations [9,10,15–17]. A systematic review by Krause et al. presents evidence that HIVST is highly acceptable among key populations [8]. In Rwanda, a qualitative study on men's perspectives towards HIVST revealed that men found HIVST acceptable; however, lack of awareness, cost of the kits, and concerns over potential social harm and possible adverse events were reported as potential barriers to uptake [18].

With a goal to end AIDS by 2030 [19,20]; this goal calls for strategic implementation and scale-up strategies that result in increased uptake HTS. Within SSA Africa, Kenya has effectively implemented guidelines on programmatic approaches to HIVST. The Kenyan guidelines for HIVST describe the package of support services, commodity management systems, the coordination mechanisms, quality assurance measures, and describing some of the monitoring and evaluation strategies [21]. These guidelines played a key role in ensuring effective implementation and scale-up of HIVST in Kenya. The relevance of stakeholders in the implementation of policies in every healthcare delivery cannot be over-emphasized. Evidence has demonstrated the important role of stakeholders in the successful implementation of health policies [22,23]. The implementation and scale-up efforts for HIVST in Rwanda will rely largely on informed strategies that ensure improved uptake [24]. Adequate involvement of all the relevant stakeholders is crucial for the overall success of the implementation and scale-up efforts. This study therefore sought to explore the perspectives of key stakeholders concerning the implementation and scale-up of HIVST in Rwanda.

2. Materials and Methods

This study was conducted as part of a large study entitled: Adaptation of a Health Education Program for Improving Uptake of HIV Self-Testing among Men in Rwanda. The protocol for the main study is under consideration for publication elsewhere.

2.1. Ethics

This study has been ethically reviewed and approved by four institutional review boards: the Rwanda National Ethics Committee (Approval number: 332/RNEC/201; May 29th 2019), University Teaching Hospital of Kigali Ethics Committee (Approval number: EC/CHUK/0111/2019; June 17th 2019), Rwanda Military Hospital Institutional Review Board (Approval number: RMH IRB/036/2019; July 12th 2019) and the University of KwaZulu Natal Biomedical Research Ethics Committee (Approval number: BE/280/19; June 24th 2019). Study participants were provided with an information sheet explaining the objectives of the study, and all participants signed informed consent forms prior to participation.

2.2. Study Setting

Kigali Province is the capital city of Rwanda. It consists of three Districts, namely Gasabo, Kicukiro and Nyarugenge, 35 sectors, 161 cells, and 1183 villages in Kigali [25]. Kigali City houses all national-level stakeholders in the HIV program in Rwanda [26]. The overall HIV prevalence among adults in Rwanda is 3.0% [2]. Annual incidence of HIV among adults (defined as those aged 15–64 years) in Rwanda was 0.08% [2]. This corresponds to approximately 5,400 new cases of HIV annually among adults in Rwanda [2]. With a goal to end AIDS by 2030 [26], Rwanda is intensifying evidence-based interventions such as HIVST to further reduce HIV incidence.

2.3. Study Sample

In the study, the sample consisted of 13 purposively-selected key stakeholders. In particular, the sample was drawn from the Ministry of Health, Rwanda Biomedical Center, non-governmental organizations and HIV clinics at tertiary health facilities in Kigali.

2.4. Data Collection

We collected qualitative data from the key stakeholders using in-depth interviews. Interviews were conducted by trained researchers using an interview guide (Supplementary File 1), which contained open-ended questions. Interviews were conducted between September 2019 and November 2019 in different settings where the stakeholders or public health officials serve. Interviews were conducted in English and in Kinyarwanda languages and continued until saturation was reached; when no additional information was emerging from the interviews [27]. Interviews conducted in Kinyarwanda were translated by a professional translator with back translation to ensure no loss of data.

2.5. Data Entry and Analysis

The interviews conducted were audio-recorded and transcribed verbatim in Microsoft Word 2016. Verbatim transcription of all interviews, with study participant's checking [27] to seek points of clarification in relation to issues arising from interviews, was performed to ensure the validity of the interviews. All interview transcripts were uploaded into NVivo v12 software (QSR International Pty Ltd., Melbourne, Australia) for analysis. Framework-based thematic analysis was performed by TD and CK, in parallel guided by the Consolidated Framework for Implementation Research (CFIR) [28]. The framework-based synthesis approach followed these steps: familiarization; identifying a thematic framework; indexing; charting; and mapping and interpretation. This approach has been applied in policy-related research questions [29]. This approach enabled domains identified in advance in the CFIR to be explicitly and systematically considered in the analysis, while also facilitating enough flexibility to detect and characterise issues that emerged from the transcripts [30]. First, the authors familiarized themselves with the content of the transcripts. Secondly, participants' responses were coded into categories based on the CFIR domains, which were then grouped into nodes. Using the relationships module of NVivo, the nodes were grouped into similar concepts that reflect key stakeholders' perspectives on implementation and scale-up of HIVST in Rwanda. Finally, mapping and interpretation of the themes and sub-themes was done.

3. Results

In total, we interviewed 13 participants, including HIVST key stakeholders in Rwanda's HIV programs. In this study, we defined HIVST stakeholders as professionals working within the Rwanda Ministry of Health and its partners responsible for the implementation of HIVST in Rwanda. The individuals formed part of the national-level technical working group for HIVST implementation with oversight of implementation and scale-up efforts nationally. The characteristics of study participants are outlined in Table 1.

Table 1. The presentation of key stakeholders by age, gender, highest qualification, number of years' experience in the HIV response and role in HIVST implementation in Rwanda.

Participant ID	Age	Gender	Education Level	Years' Experience in the HIV Response in Rwanda	Role in HIVST Implementation
#1	40	Female	Undergraduate	13	Program Manager, Policy maker
#2	30	Male	Undergraduate	5	Health care provider, policy maker
#3	41	Male	Undergraduate	10	Program Manager, Policy maker
#4	45	Male	Post-graduate	15	Program Manager, Policy maker
#5	42	Female	Post-graduate	15	Program Manager, Policy maker
#6	33	Male	Undergraduate	11	Supply Chain Specialist, Policy advisor
#7	29	Female	Undergraduate	5	Health care provider, policy maker
#8	44	Male	Doctorate	15	Researcher, Stakeholder
#9	50	Male	Doctorate	25	Researcher, Stakeholder
#10	48	Male	Undergraduate	15	Health care provider, policy maker
#11	49	Male	Post-graduate	15	Health care provider, policy maker
#12	37	Male	Doctorate	8	Laboratory Specialist, Policy maker
#13	39	Male	Doctorate	16	Researcher, Stakeholder

Key stakeholders were all well-aware of HIVST intervention and perceived HIVST as a potentially-effective initiative which can be used in order to ensure that there is improvement in uptake of testing services, especially for underserved populations in Rwanda.

3.1. Researcher, Stakeholder

"HIV self-testing basically refers to the process through which an individual who is interested in knowing their HIV status carry out the HIV test by themselves. They also interpret the result in private. It is just one of the ways through which individuals can get to know their HIV status after buying the self-test kits. It was introduced in order to address the challenges of stigma and confidentiality associated with routine provider initiated or voluntary counseling and testing. It offers the potential for HIV testing to reach more people than previously possible, including those who do not seek testing in our health facilities here".

3.2. Supply Chain Specialist, Policy Advisor

"It is an additional or a new approach in Rwanda to boost the existing HIV testing services that we currently have. It is a screening test which detects HIV antibodies. Currently in our country, it is in the pilot phase, not yet well implemented in the whole country. We have kits distributed in different pharmacies in Kigali and those vendors explain to those who come to buy it on how they can use it accordingly".

4. Emerging Themes

Three main themes emerged: HIVST is a potentially effective initiative to improve uptake of HIV testing services; challenges hindering effective implementation; and potential strategies which can be adopted to ensure effective implementation and scale-up of HIVST. The emerging themes and sub-themes are presented in Table 2.

Table 2. Themes and sub-themes.

THEMES	SUB-THEME(S)
Theme 1: Potentially effective initiative to improve uptake of HIV testing services	• Target people unwilling to use facility-based testing services
Theme 2: Challenges hindering implementation and scale up of HIVST	• Poor awareness • High cost of the kits • Concerns on results interpretation
Theme 3: Strategies to improve implementation and scale up	• Creation of awareness/knowledge of the intervention • Training those involved in implementation • Regulation of sell of self-test kits • Reducing the costs of the kits through the provision of subsidies • Ensure consistent availability of the self-test kits.

A detailed framework analysis of key stakeholders' responses guided by the CFIR is presented on Supplemental File 2.

4.1. Theme 1

Key stakeholders perceived HIVST as an acceptable intervention with the potential to bridge the gap in the uptake of HTS. In addition to the general population, most stakeholders listed men, female sex workers, men who have sex with men, and the rick/famous people as potential groups that could benefit from HIVST initiative in Rwanda.

4.1.1. Program Manager, Policy Maker

"Thank you, so (HIV) self-testing is one of the approaches that we are using to make sure that people know their HIV status. It was started as an additional option for people who want to know their HIV status and especially those who are not willing to use conventional HIV testing methods which are facility-based. This was chosen as an approach that will be increasing the number of people who are aware of their HIV status".

4.1.2. Researcher, Stakeholder

"I think it (HIVST) is a noble intervention, which will play a key role in ensuring that there is an improvement in the uptake of HIV testing services, more so among the people who are otherwise normally hard to reach. It comes with a number of advantages, which generally include privacy, convenience, confidentiality, and ease of use".

4.1.3. Program Manager, Policy Maker

"HIV testing services are available, free of charge, and available to all public health facilities, but we have some groups who don't reach those services for their own reasons, maybe self-stigma in the case of sex workers, maybe being too busy like men, or they are rich and famous. All these groups can now access [HIV] self-testing".

4.1.4. Laboratory Specialist, Policy Maker

"Currently, we have only one kit available on the local market and at health facilities. OraQuick (manufactured) by Orasure Technologies. We performed in-house validations here at the reference lab. We obtained over 90% sensitivity for oral fluid. So as (HIV) program, we are confident this test can help improve our numbers on the first 90. More people can now get tested and interpret their own results. The only caveat is those results are not final; patients would still need to visit a health facility for retesting and confirmation".

4.2. Theme 2: Challenges Hindering Implementation and Scale up of HIVST

Key stakeholders alluded to challenges that were impeding the implementation and scale-up of HIVST in Rwanda. The participants presented a mix of intervention characteristics, outer and inner settings challenges. Most participants strongly felt the need to prioritize addressing these challenges before efforts to implement and scale-up HIVST are commenced in Rwanda.

4.2.1. Sub Theme 1: Lack of Awareness

A general lack of awareness among the users of the kits emerged as a sub-theme. Stakeholders noted some concerns relating to lack of awareness of/on HIVST among the general population. Further, stakeholders noted that HIVST is still inaccessible to rural populations that are also resource-limited in terms of health facilities. Key stakeholders perceived that not much awareness has been created. They also noted that some of the people with access to the kits do not have adequate levels of education and knowledge on how to use them.

4.2.2. Researcher, Stakeholder

"Before the government decides to ensure that it is rolled up on a large scale, I think they need to ensure that people are aware of the kits. At the moment I think that not so many people know about them. Again, the government should work on the costs that are associated with the acquisition of the kits. At the moment, it is beyond the reach of most of the people who are the main targets."

4.2.3. Sub Theme 2: Cost of the Kits

Key informants perceived the costs of purchasing the kits as one of the main barriers to the effective implementation and scale-up of HIVST in Rwanda.

4.2.4. Health Care Provider, Policy Maker

"I think that the ministry of health is still facing different kinds of challenges, which needs to be addressed to ensure effective implementation of self-testing. For instance, the general lack of the guidance on HIV self-testing, and the lack of low-cost test kits and the systems to assess and regulate them, have been a key barrier to implementation. They need to be addressed effectively. The ministry of health should also adopt policy guidelines that inform the adoption of suitable HIVST test kits, taking into consideration who exactly we want to get tested."

4.2.5. Sub Theme 3: Results Interpretation

Key stakeholders noted their concerns on the interpretation of results following HIVST testing. Key stakeholders were of the perspective that reported cases of discordant results between the HIV self-test and repeat testing at a health facility were mainly user-based. Issues with the interpretation of results were revealed as key in these discrepancies.

4.2.6. Program Manager, Policy Maker

"HIV self-testing is very new in Rwanda. So far, I only can think of two challenges. For instance, we have received cases of false positives and negatives. This creates a problem. Even though the cases are few, it is enough to raise concern as it may affect uptake. Once a bad message is passed about HIV self-testing giving incorrect results, it may lower uptake significantly. And we don't want that. (...) Basically, it comes down to ensuring those that are selling in private pharmacies or distributing at our (government) facilities are trained so they can train the users and the issue of regulation of sale of these self-test kits."

4.3. Theme 3: Strategies to Improve Implementation and Scale-up of HIVST in Rwanda

Key stakeholders presented their views on strategies which can be used to ensure successful implementation and scale-up of HIVST. These include the following: the creation of awareness; training those involved in the implementation process; regulation of the selling of the self-test kits; reduction of the costs of acquiring the self-test kits through the provision of subsidies; and ensuring consistent availability of the self-test kits.

4.3.1. Sub Theme 1: Creation of Awareness

The need for the creation of awareness on HIVST in order to ensure uptake was noted by most key stakeholders. Community mobilization strategies proposed by some stakeholders include decentralized campaigns, community-led advocacy through the monthly *umuganda* community meetings, and radio jingles.

4.3.2. Supply Chain Specialist, Policy Advisor

"The uptake of HIV self-testing is still very low, and as you may be aware, not much has been done to ensure that it is available to all the people in Rwanda, including those in the remote areas. So far, the focus has been only in Kigali City. There are also people who are still not aware of HIV self-testing. The government, therefore, needs to do much more to ensure that more people are made to be aware of HIV self-testing".

4.3.3. Program Manager, Policy Maker

"I recommend improving awareness, to encourage those groups who don't get HIV testing and then to make availability of test kits at a low price."

4.3.4. Sub Theme 2: Training of the People Involved in the Implementation Process

Key stakeholders emphasized the need for providing training to all parties involved in the implementation of the HIVST intervention in order to ensure successful implementation.

4.3.5. Health Care Provider, Stakeholder

"The government should just ensure that it (implementation) is done in the right manner by training all the people involved, doing mass campaigns to ensure that more people are aware of the existence of the programs, and ensuring that there are proper distribution channels of the HIV (self) test kits".

4.3.6. Sub Theme 3: Proper Regulation of the Kits

A common theme, on the strategies to ensure effective implementation and scale-up of HIVST implementation, was the need to ensure proper regulation of the self-test kits. Stakeholders noted that currently in Rwanda HIV self-test kits are available for purchase online. Stakeholders perceived the need for ensuring guidelines are followed with regard to certification for use of these kits.

4.3.7. Laboratory Specialist, Policy Maker

"I also believe that proper regulation can play a key role in ensuring that some of the key challenges I have discussed earlier are addressed. We validated for use in Rwanda the test kits currently in circulation. We are also involved in ensuring quality assurance for new kit lots and surveillance for cases of false positive or negative results. We monitor those as well."

4.3.8. Sub Theme 4: Reducing the Costs of the Kits

Most of the stakeholders were of the viewpoint that the kits are currently going for 5000 RWF for one test, which is not within the reach of most of the people who are targeted. As a result, effective implementation and scale-up of the kits needs measures to be put in place to subsidize the costs of acquiring the kits. This will make the kits to be within the reach of the users.

4.3.9. Researcher, Stakeholder

"I think the ministry should look at the processes that are currently being charged. The kit currently costs 5000 Rwandan Francs in pharmacies in Rwanda and I think this is too expensive. While the government is working to ensure that the kits are available in the entire country, they need to ensure that there are measures aimed at lowering the prices of the kits. For such an important intervention, it is reasonable to provide subsidies to cushion users".

4.3.10. Sub Theme 5: Ensuring Availability of the Kits

When it comes to effective implementation and scale-up of HIVST, key stakeholders perceived the need for the government of Rwanda to ensure that there are measures in place to ensure constant availability of kits. This means ensuring the availability of stock and proper distribution channels to improve uptake.

4.3.11. Program Manager, Policy Maker

"I think here the most important point is to see how we can increase kit availability by ensuring adequate stock levels at MPPD always, and appropriate space where the kits will be distributed. So far, we have them limited at pharmacies, a few health facilities and online purchases. To improve uptake when we scale-up, there is a need to have a wider range of distribution channels".

5. Discussion

This study presents perceptions of HIVST key stakeholders on the implementation and scale-up of HIVST in Rwanda. Key stakeholders perceive HIVST to be a highly effective intervention for helping the underserved populations access HTS. This corroborates well with WHO recommendations on HIVST as an additional strategy to improve uptake of HTS [5]. Interventions aimed at improving uptake of HTS as an important step to attaining the UNAIDS 90-90-90 target of 2020 have been underscored in the Rwanda 2019–2024 Fourth Health Sector Strategic Plan [26]. Our findings reveal that key stakeholders perceive HIVST as an important gateway to realization of the UNAIDS 90-90-90 targets. Theme two identified key stakeholders' perceived challenges for implementation and scale-up of HIVST; lack of awareness of the kits, high cost of the self-test kits, and concerns over results interpretation. Low awareness was mainly attributed to the intervention being relatively new in Rwanda and still in pilot phases. Theme three: key stakeholders' perceived measures of what is necessary for the successful implementation and scale-up of HIVST in Rwanda included the creation of awareness, training those involved in the implementation process, regulation of the selling of the self-test kits, reduction of the costs of acquiring the self-test kits, and ensuring consistent availability of the self-test kits. Health education programs, community mobilization, development of HIVST country guidelines and provision of subsidies to cushion the cost of test kits would strengthen implementation and scale-up efforts for HIVST in Rwanda.

In the current study, key stakeholders' perceived HIVST as an auspicious intervention with the potential to bridge the current gap in uptake of HTS in Rwanda. This corroborates well with findings from a similar study conducted in South Africa, which demonstrated key stakeholders' confidence in HIVST improving uptake of HTS in underserved population [31]. A recently published systematic review and meta-synthesis on men's perspectives on HIV self-testing in sub-Saharan Africa recommended presented evidence of poor awareness but high acceptability of HIVST among men [32]. While this is the case; stakeholders expressed concerns that need to be addressed before effective implementation and scale-up can be achieved. Concerns cited by key stakeholders in the current study on the regulation of the sale of test-kits and results interpretation have been reported elsewhere [7,33–35]. Healthcare workers in Kenya concerned with challenges with test results interpretation recommended proper regulatory measures to be put in place prior to scale of HIVST intervention [7]. Similarly, healthcare providers in Kwa-Zulu Natal province in South Africa perceived issues with results interpretation as a potential challenge with HIVST implementation in South Africa [33]. A cross-sectional study on participants without prior experience with the HIV self-test revealed the most common interpretation error was incorrectly identifying a negative result as invalid [10]. Raising public awareness levels emerged as a key strategy to effective implementation and overall success of scale-up efforts in this study. Similar recommendations have been made elsewhere [31,32,36,37]. Key stakeholders in South Africa [31], researchers, academics, journalists, community advocates, policy makers and other key stakeholders in Nigeria [36] and reviews by Hlongwa et al. [32], Johnson et al. [37] all recommend need the improve public awareness on HIVST. Similar to the findings of the current study, ensuring that kits are affordable has been recommended by key stakeholders in South Africa [31,33] and potential users in Singapore [10].

The study has demonstrated the feasibility of HIVST implementation and scale-up in Rwanda from a key stakeholder's perspective. There is a need to document HIVST guidelines and policies that define the supply chain, stakeholder roles and responsibilities, implementation strategy, quality assurance measures, and monitoring and evaluation strategies. Policymakers need to ensure that effective mobilization programs are designed to raise public awareness. Training for those involved in the implementation and subsequent step-down training will be key in the implementation and scale-up efforts of HIVST in Rwanda.

A notable strength of the current study is that the majority of the key stakeholders were men. The current study is part of a larger study aimed at adaptation of a health education program for improving the uptake of HIVST among men. A limitation of this study was that only national-level key stakeholders residing in Kigali were enrolled, thus limiting the generalization of study findings to other settings. There is a need for further research incorporating lower-level stakeholders and to fully understand the challenges and inform policy. However, our sample was drawn from individuals who are responsible for the implementation of HIVST in the country, with knowledge on the status of the current implementation and scale-up efforts across the country. Finally, qualitative findings are highly subjective [38]. However, we used prolonged engagement [39,40] to ensure credibility and pilot testing of the interview guide [41,42] to ensure dependability. We enhanced the credibility and dependability of the study findings by following a rigorous inductive analysis and interpretation of the data. We also employed note-taking [42] and participant validation of transcripts [43] to enhance the credibility of the reported findings.

6. Conclusions

The current study findings demonstrate the confidence of key stakeholders in the Rwanda health system to effectively sustain the HIVST intervention. The concerns raised over factors with the potential to impede smooth implementation and scale-up should be addressed.

Supplementary Materials: The following are available online at http://www.mdpi.com/2075-4418/10/4/194/s1, Supplementary File 1: Interview guides for the in-depth interviews with different key stakeholders and health care providers. Supplemental File 2: Detailed analysis of the interview transcripts against the Consolidated Framework for Implementation Research.

Author Contributions: T.D. and T.P.M.-T. conceptualized the study. T.D. and C.K. carried out the first analysis of the study. T.D. produced the first draft of the manuscript. T.P.M.-T. reviewed the draft and contributed to the final version. All authors have read and agreed to the published version of the manuscript.

Funding: The University of KwaZulu-Natal, College of Health Sciences PhD Scholarship supported this study (Grant number 641581). The funder had no role in study design, data collection and analysis, decision to publish, or preparation of the manuscript.

Acknowledgments: The authors would like to thank all stakeholders that participated in this study by sharing their valuable input. Tafadzwa Dzinamarira is supported by The University of KwaZulu-Natal, College of Health Sciences PhD Scholarship. This study was supported by the CIHR Canadian HIV Trials Network (CTN 222). Tivani P. Mashamba-Thompson is supported by CTN Postdoctoral Fellowship Award. The funders had no role in study design, data collection and analysis, decision to publish, or preparation of the manuscript. Further, the authors acknowledge Claude Mambo Muvunyi and Gashema Pierre for their contribution in the data analysis.

Conflicts of Interest: The authors declare no conflict of interest.

References

1. WHO. HIV Self-Testing. 2019. Available online: https://www.who.int/hiv/topics/self-testing/en/ (accessed on 30 November 2019).
2. ICAP. Summary Sheet: Preliminary Findings: Rwanda Population-Based HIV Impact Assessment RPHIA 2018–2019. 2019. Available online: https://phia.icap.columbia.edu/wp-content/uploads/2019/10/RPHIA-Summary-Sheet_Oct-2019.pdf (accessed on 2 December 2019).
3. Johnson, C.C.; Kennedy, C.; Fonner, V.; Siegfried, N.; Figueroa, C.; Dalal, S.; Sands, A.; Baggaley, R. Examining the effects of HIV self-testing compared to standard HIV testing services: A systematic review and meta-analysis. *J. Int AIDS Soc.* **2017**, *20*, 21594. [CrossRef]
4. El-Sadr, W.M.; Harripersaud, K.; Rabkin, M. Reaching global HIV/AIDS goals: What got us here, won't get us there. *PLoS Med.* **2017**, *14*, e1002421. [CrossRef]
5. WHO. *Guidelines on HIV Self-Testing and Partner Notification: Supplement to Consolidated Guidelines on HIV Testing Services*; 9241549866; World Health Organization: Geneva, Switzerland, 2016.
6. MOH. *Strategic Plans*; Moh.gov.rw; MOH: Kigali, Rwanda, 2019.
7. Kalibala, S.; Tun, W.; Cherutich, P.; Nganga, A.; Oweya, E.; Oluoch, P. Factors associated with acceptability of HIV self-testing among health care workers in Kenya. *Aids Behav.* **2014**, *18*, 405–414. [CrossRef]
8. Krause, J.; Subklew-Sehume, F.; Kenyon, C.; Colebunders, R. Acceptability of HIV self-testing: A systematic literature review. *Bmc Public Health.* **2013**, *13*, 735. [CrossRef] [PubMed]
9. Volk, J.E.; Lippman, S.A.; Grinsztejn, B.; Lama, J.R.; Fernandes, N.M.; Gonzales, P.; Hessol, N.A.; Buchbinder, S. Acceptability and feasibility of HIV self-testing among men who have sex with men in Peru and Brazil. *Int. J. Std Aids* **2016**, *27*, 531–536. [CrossRef] [PubMed]
10. Ng, O.T.; Chow, A.L.; Lee, V.J.; Chen, M.I.; Win, M.K.; Tan, H.H.; Chua, A.; Leo, Y.S. Accuracy and user-acceptability of HIV self-testing using an oral fluid-based HIV rapid test. *PLoS ONE* **2012**, *7*, e45168. [CrossRef] [PubMed]
11. Kurth, A.E.; Cleland, C.M.; Chhun, N.; Sidle, J.E.; Were, E.; Naanyu, V.; Emonyi, W.; Macharia, S.M.; Sang, E.; Siika, A.M. Accuracy and acceptability of oral fluid HIV self-testing in a general adult population in Kenya. *Aids Behav.* **2016**, *20*, 870–879. [CrossRef]
12. Van Dyk, A.C. Client-initiated, provider-initiated, or self-testing for HIV: What do South Africans prefer? *J. Assoc. Nurses Aids Care* **2013**, *24*, e45–e56. [CrossRef]
13. Wong, H.T.H.; Tam, H.Y.; Chan, D.P.C.; Lee, S.S.J. Usage and acceptability of HIV self-testing in men who have sex with men in Hong Kong. *Aids Behav.* **2015**, *19*, 505–515. [CrossRef] [PubMed]
14. Izizag, B.B.; Situakibanza, H.; Mbutiwi, T.; Ingwe, R.; Kiazayawoko, F.; Nkodila, A.; Mandina, M.; Longokolo, M.; Amaela, E.; Mbula, M. Factors associated with acceptability of HIV self-testing (HIVST) among university students in a Peri-Urban area of the Democratic Republic of Congo (DRC). *Pan Afr. Med. J.* **2018**, *31*, 248. [CrossRef]

15. Marlin, R.W.; Young, S.D.; Bristow, C.C.; Wilson, G.; Rodriguez, J.; Ortiz, J.; Mathew, R.; Klausner, J.D. Piloting an HIV self-test kit voucher program to raise serostatus awareness of high-risk African Americans, Los Angeles. *Bmc Public Health* **2014**, *14*, 1226. [CrossRef] [PubMed]
16. Heard, A.C.; Brown, A.N. Public readiness for HIV self-testing in Kenya. *Aids Care* **2016**, *28*, 1528–1532. [CrossRef] [PubMed]
17. Harichund, C.; Moshabela, M.; Kunene, P.; Abdool Karim, Q. Acceptability of HIV self-testing among men and women in KwaZulu-Natal, South Africa. *Aids Care* **2019**, *31*, 186–192. [CrossRef] [PubMed]
18. Dzinamarira, T.; Pierre, G.; Rujeni, N. Is HIV Self-Testing a Potential Answer to the Low Uptake of HIV Testing Services Among Men in Rwanda? Perspectives of Men Attending Tertiary Institutions and Kimisagara Youth Centre in Kigali, Rwanda. *Glob. J. Health Sci.* **2019**, *11*, 67. [CrossRef]
19. WHO. *End HIV/AIDS by 2030; HIV/AIDS: Framework for Action in the WHO African Region, 2016–2020*; WHO: Geneva, Switzerland, 2019.
20. UNAIDS. Fast-Track Commitments to End Aids by 2030. 2019. Available online: https://www.unaids.org/sites/default/files/media_asset/fast-track-commitments_en.pdf (accessed on 4 December 2019).
21. NASCOP. *HIV Self-Testing: An Operational Manual for the Delivery of HIV Self-Testing Services in Kenya*; NASCOP: Nairobi, Kenya, 2017.
22. Aniteye, P.; Mayhew, S.H. Shaping legal abortion provision in Ghana: Using policy theory to understand provider-related obstacles to policy implementation. *Health Res. Policy Syst.* **2013**, *11*, 23. [CrossRef]
23. Bennett, S.; Mahmood, S.S.; Edward, A.; Tetui, M.; Ekirapa-Kiracho, E. Strengthening scaling up through learning from implementation: Comparing experiences from Afghanistan, Bangladesh and Uganda. *Health Res. Policy Syst.* **2017**, *15*, 108. [CrossRef]
24. Dzinamarira, T. The Call to Get More Men Tested for HIV: A Perspective on What Policy Makers Need to Know for Implementing and Scaling up HIV Self-Testing in Rwanda. *Glob. J. Health Sci.* **2019**, *11*. [CrossRef]
25. NISR, M. *Rwanda Fourth Population and Housing Census 2012. Thematic Report on Population Size, Structure and Distribution*; NISR: Kigali, Rwanda, 2014.
26. Health, M.O. *Fourth Health Sector Strategic Plan July 2018–June 2024*; MOH: Kigali, Rwanda, 2018.
27. Saunders, B.; Sim, J.; Kingstone, T.; Baker, S.; Waterfield, J.; Bartlam, B.; Burroughs, H.; Jinks, C. Saturation in qualitative research: Exploring its conceptualization and operationalization. *Qual Quant.* **2018**, *52*, 1893–1907. [CrossRef]
28. Damschroder, L.J.; Aron, D.C.; Keith, R.E.; Kirsh, S.R.; Alexander, J.A.; Lowery, J.C. Fostering implementation of health services research findings into practice: A consolidated framework for advancing implementation science. *Implement. Sci.* **2009**, *4*, 50. [CrossRef]
29. Wood, F.; Robling, M.; Prout, H.; Kinnersley, P.; Houston, H.; Butler, C.J.T. A question of balance: A qualitative study of mothers' interpretations of dietary recommendations. *Ann. Fam. Med.* **2010**, *8*, 51–57. [CrossRef]
30. Dixon-Woods, M.; Agarwal, S.; Jones, D.; Young, B.; Sutton, A. Synthesising qualitative and quantitative evidence: A review of possible methods. *J. Health Serv. Res. Policy* **2005**, *10*, 45–53. [CrossRef] [PubMed]
31. Makusha, T.; Knight, L.; Taegtmeyer, M.; Tulloch, O.; Davids, A.; Lim, J.; Peck, R.; van Rooyen, H. HIV self-testing could "revolutionize testing in South Africa, but it has got to be done properly": Perceptions of key stakeholders. *PLoS ONE* **2015**, *10*, e0122783. [CrossRef] [PubMed]
32. Hlongwa, M.; Mashamba-Thompson, T.; Makhunga, S.; Muraraneza, C.; Hlongwana, K. Men's perspectives on HIV self-testing in sub-Saharan Africa: A systematic review and meta-synthesis. *Bmc Public Health* **2020**, *20*, 66. [CrossRef] [PubMed]
33. Gumede, S.D.; Sibiya, M.N. Health care users' knowledge, attitudes and perceptions of HIV self-testing at selected gateway clinics at eThekwini district, KwaZulu-Natal province, South Africa. *SAHARA J.* **2018**, *15*, 103–109. [CrossRef]
34. Richter, M.; Venter, W.; Gray, A. Enabling HIV self-testing in South Africa. *S. Afr. J. Hiv Med.* **2012**, *13*, 186–187. [CrossRef]
35. Napierala Mavedzenge, S.; Baggaley, R.; Corbett, E.L. A review of self-testing for HIV: Research and policy priorities in a new era of HIV prevention. *Clin. Infect Dis.* **2013**, *57*, 126–138. [CrossRef]
36. Brown, B.; Folayan, M.O.; Imosili, A.; Durueke, F.; Amuamuziam, A. HIV self-testing in Nigeria: Public opinions and perspectives. *Glob. Public Health.* **2015**, *10*, 354–365. [CrossRef]
37. Johnson, C.; Baggaley, R.; Forsythe, S.; Van Rooyen, H.; Ford, N.; Mavedzenge, S.N.; Corbett, E.; Natarajan, P.; Taegtmeyer, M. Realizing the potential for HIV self-testing. *Aids Behav.* **2014**, *18*, 391–395. [CrossRef]

38. Queirós, A.; Faria, D.; Almeida, F. Strengths and limitations of qualitative and quantitative research methods. *Eur. J. Educ. Stud.* **2017**, *3*. [CrossRef]
39. Talbot, L. *Principles and Practice of Nursing Research*; Mosby Incorporated: St. Louis, MO, USA, 1995; p. 700.
40. Lincoln, Y.S.; Guba, E.G. Establishing trustworthiness. *Nat. Inq.* **1985**, *289*, 331.
41. Polit, D.F.; Beck, C.T. *Nursing Research: Generating and Assessing Evidence for Nursing Practice*; Lippincott Williams & Wilkins: Philadelphia, PA, USA, 2008.
42. Patton, M.Q. Enhancing the quality and credibility of qualitative analysis. *Health Serv. Res.* **1999**, *34*, 1189. [PubMed]
43. Birt, L.; Scott, S.; Cavers, D.; Campbell, C.; Walter, F. Member Checking: A Tool to Enhance Trustworthiness or Merely a Nod to Validation? *Qual. Health Res.* **2016**, *26*, 1802–1811. [CrossRef] [PubMed]

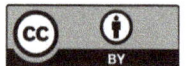

© 2020 by the authors. Licensee MDPI, Basel, Switzerland. This article is an open access article distributed under the terms and conditions of the Creative Commons Attribution (CC BY) license (http://creativecommons.org/licenses/by/4.0/).

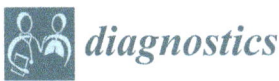

Case Report

Use of a Smartphone-Based Augmented Reality Video Conference App to Remotely Guide a Point of Care Ultrasound Examination

Davinder Ramsingh [1,*], Cori Van Gorkom [1], Matthew Holsclaw [1], Scott Nelson [2], Martin De La Huerta [2], Julian Hinson [1] and Emilie Selleck [1]

1. Department of Anesthesiology, Loma Linda University Health, 11234 Anderson Street MC-2532, Loma Linda, CA 92354, USA; CVangorkom@llu.edu (C.V.G.); mholsclaw@llu.edu (M.H.); jhinson@llu.edu (J.H.); ESelleck@llu.edu (E.S.)
2. Department of Orthopedic Surgery, Haiti Adventist Hospital, Route De La Mairie De Carrefour, Diquini 63, Haiti; scnelson@llu.edu (S.N.); Delahuertam@yahoo.com (M.D.L.H.)
* Correspondence: dramsingh@llu.edu

Received: 20 September 2019; Accepted: 22 October 2019; Published: 24 October 2019

Abstract: Reports on the use of various smartphone-based video conference applications to guide point-of-care ultrasound (POCUS) examinations in resource-limited settings have been described. However, the use of an augmented reality-enabled smartphone video conference application in this same manner has not been described. Presented is a case in which such as application was used to remotely guide a point of care ultrasound examination.

Keywords: point of care ultrasound; augmented reality; telemedicine

1. Introduction

The ability to improve the quality of care to resource-limited settings is often a logistical challenge resulting from the lack of specialized medical practitioners and services. This is often secondary to geographic, demographic, and socioeconomic factors. The implementation of technology in healthcare is often a contributor to this problem rather than a solution. However, recent innovations in smartphone technology and point-of-care ultrasound (POCUS) devices have proven to be key examples of how technological advances are poised to elevate the quality of care in resource-limited settings. Indeed, the use of smartphone devices to provide real-time video conferences has proven to improve rural medicine across many medical specialties [1–5]. Similarly, the advancements in POCUS technology have greatly facilitated the ability to perform ultrasound exams in remote patient care settings.

Point-of-care ultrasound refers to the use of ultrasonography at the patient's bedside for diagnostic and therapeutic purposes [6]. The provider acquires and interprets all images in real-time and then uses that information to diagnose and direct therapies. Of note, POCUS has been identified as the most rapidly growing sector in medical ultrasound imaging [7]. Recent advances in this technology include improved image quality as well as a significant reduction in price, with handheld devices costing approximately 1/20th the price of devices ten years ago (from USD 40,000+ to USD 2000).

Recently, smartphone-based video conference technologies have been used with point-of-care ultrasound. Several studies have demonstrated the ability to remotely educate, guide, and provide image interpretation of POCUS examinations. While these studies have shown promise, a new modality, augmented reality (AR), has recently been implemented in the point-of-care ultrasound education space [8]. The use of AR has demonstrated utility in the remote guidance of POCUS [8]. However, the use of AR to improve remote medical training has mostly been described with the use of specialized equipment that may not be readily available in resource-limited environments.

This report highlights the use of a novel smartphone application (Vuforia Chalk, San Diego CA, USA) to provide AR remote assistance to guide a POCUS examination. The application works on most smartphone devices and web browsers and provides an augmented reality video conference interface that allows each user to notate the other's environment (see Figure 1). The ease of use and widespread applicability across multiple smartphone platforms allows this program to potentially improve the availability of remote AR guidance to teach POCUS in resource-limited settings. This non-sponsored case report was a proof-of-concept evaluation on the feasibility of using this AR application to improve remote guidance of POCUS examinations in a resource-limited environment. Specialty-trained providers from a tertiary care center, Loma Linda University Medical Center (LLUMC), in California, USA, successfully used this application to provide remote AR guidance for a POCUS examination at a rural hospital in Port-au-Prince, Haiti.

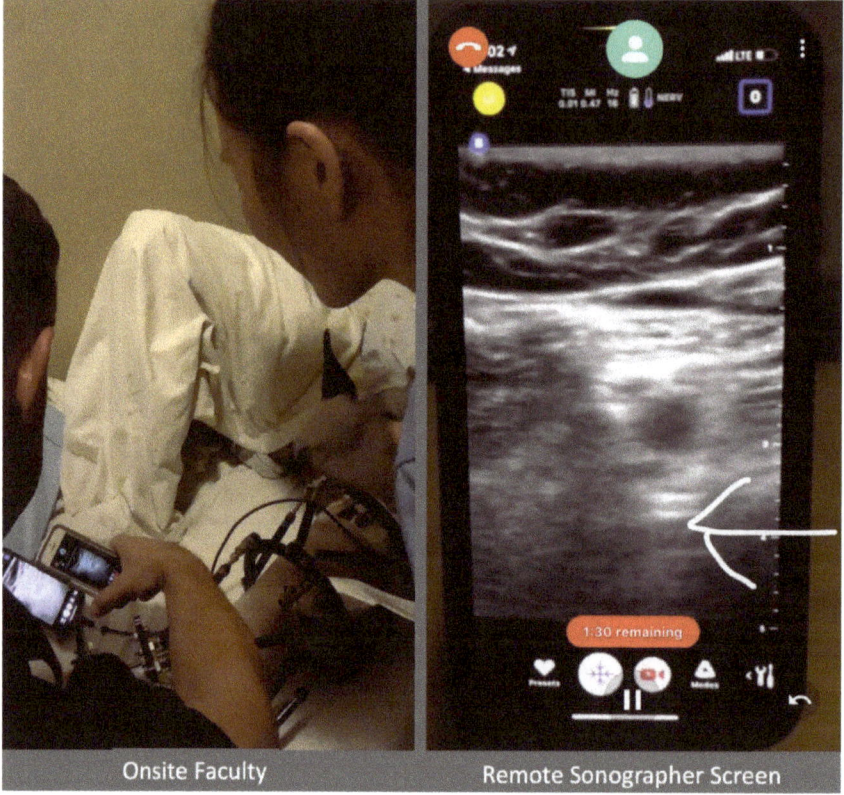

Figure 1. Overview of Onsite and Remote Augmented Reality Enhanced Video Communication. The white arrow indicates the femur, which was identified for anatomy review during remote guidance communication.

2. Description of the Case

Faculty from the tertiary care center traveled with a low-cost ($2000 USD) handheld portable ultrasound device (Butterfly Network, Guilford, CT. USA) and a *Chalk*-enabled smartphone (iPhone 8, Apple Cupertino, CA. USA) to the Hôpital Adventiste d'Haiti. During the visit, the onsite and visiting faculty identified a 35-year-old male patient scheduled to undergo an external fixator removal and replacement. The patient required a regional anesthesia popliteal nerve block. The ability to use ultrasound to perform this block was not routinely available, and local providers had not been trained to perform this procedure. To evaluate the capability of the AR application to provide remote guidance for this procedure a connection was established, via the *Chalk* application, between the visiting faculty's smartphone in Port-au-Prince, Haiti to a remote faculty in CA, USA. Consent was obtained from the patient to report this case.

The connection was established over a mobile 4g hotspot via an iPhone 5 (Apple Cupertino, CA, USA) provided by the onsite faculty. *Chalk* was used to send a call to the expert ultrasonographer (San Diego, CA, USA), who then used the AR platform to guide probe placement on the patient to obtain the appropriate ultrasound image. Once the onsite examiner had obtained the appropriate probe position and ultrasound image, the smartphone camera was adjusted to visualize the ultrasound image from the POCUS device. Specifically, the smartphone POCUS exam was placed on the patient's bed in-between their legs and the second smartphone with the AR platform was held over this device such that the ultrasound image and the AR notations could be visualized by the physician performing the exam (Figure 1). Importantly the user holding the smartphone with the AR platform was not the same person performing the procedure and would adjust the smartphone position to allow appropriate visualization for the proceduralist. The remote expert then highlighted relevant anatomy and identified the nerve on the ultrasound image via the AR platform.

The procedure was performed successfully, and the nerve block demonstrated appropriate efficacy. After the procedure, the one onsite and the one remote provider completed a survey on the image quality of the video connection. In addition, the remote provider completed a survey of the image quality of the ultrasound image viewed from the video conference app and the onsite provider completed a survey of the AR notations created by the remote provider during the guidance of the nerve block. All surveys were scored using a validated 5-point Likert scale [9].

Survey results showed that the image quality of the video communication was rated 5/5 for both video communication and ultrasound image interpretation by the one onsite and one remote practitioner. The onsite practitioner scored the clarity of the AR notations to identify probe placement position on the body as 5/5 and identification of anatomy and nerve on the ultrasound image as 4/5.

3. Discussion

Technologic advances in medical ultrasound imaging are helping remove the barriers of costs and portability. These innovations are improving the ability to use medical ultrasound in resource-limited settings as a point of care device. However, a barrier that remains is the skill/training of the providers in these settings. Programs to teach POCUS, in-person, have demonstrated to be effective [10], but have a high cost and can be difficult to repeat/grow. The use of real-time video conferencing has demonstrated to be effective for remote POCUS guidance and training [11,12]. The application of such a remote guidance and telecommunication system has demonstrated a positive clinical impact. Kolbe et al. reported a change in management in 48% of patients in a rural village in Nicaragua after the implementation of a remote guidance and telecommunication system between expert sonographers around the world and local practitioners [13]. The application of smartphone-based video conference platforms also has proven clinical utility [12]. Robertson et al. demonstrated successful communication between intensivists at a tertiary care center and non-physician health care providers in a low-income country, which demonstrated successful ability to both educate POCUS image acquisition techniques as well as allow for appropriate image quality for remote clinical interpretation [14].

In recent years, the development of AR has also been applied to POCUS. Wang et al. evaluated the feasibility of using a specific AR hardware/software platform, Microsoft HoloLens (Redmond, WA, USA), to remotely guide novice medical trainers through a trauma ultrasound examination [8]. While this does offer a tremendous opportunity to expand POCUS education, it may be less impactful in resource-limited environments. Advances in smartphone applications now allow for the use of real-time AR enhanced video communication without the need for expensive hardware. This potentially has broad implications in resource-limited areas by improving the ability to provide remote

POCUS education/guidance with low-cost smartphone and POCUS devices. While a limited example, this case demonstrates how these devices can be implemented to provide improved bedside assessment and therapies in a resource-limited environment.

Our report demonstrates the use of a smartphone app that allows for the creation of a real-time augmented reality environment in a manner very similar to common smartphone video conference applications. This proof-of-concept case report presents positive feedback from all of the providers involved and supports further exploration in this area. Of note, none of the onsite physicians involved in the case had used the Chalk app before this event. Additional discussion after the event between the onsite and remote providers highlighted that the use of this platform was an improvement over traditional smartphone video conferencing by allowing both users to provide real-time visual cues over the ultrasound image during the procedure. In addition, the AR interface provided a greater ability for depth perception compared to traditional smartphone video conferencing.

Importantly, there are several limitations for the setup described in this report. While providers reported no issues with screen glare, the use of two mobile devices to achieve the AR guidance resulted in a limitation of the field-of-view of the remote examiner. In addition, the setup described requires another individual to hold and manipulate the AR smartphone. Additionally, the placement of the ultrasound and AR devices will be different based on patient position and care setting. Finally, the AR video communication in this case report did not include the transfer of any protected health information, as this requires secure communication pathways, which have previously been described [15]. Truly, applications such as the one described in this report would require the development of these securities to provide the maximum benefit. Future evaluations of these technologies should seek to address each of these items.

Indeed, the potential widespread availability of a smartphone-based augmented reality training/guidance application makes this platform very exciting for improving healthcare in resource-limited environments by potentially providing a higher level of communication than standard video conferencing. It is the authors' hope that this report can be an example to stimulate formal research in this area.

Author Contributions: Conceptualization, D.R., and M.D.L.H.; methodology, D.R., C.V.G., M.D.L.H., S.N., M.H. and E.S.; formal analysis, D.R., J.H. and C.V.G.; software, D.R. and M.D.L.H.; investigation, D.R., C.V.G., M.D.L.H., S.N., J.H., M.D.L.H. and E.S.; writing, D.R., C.V.G., S.N., J.H., E.S.; project administration, D.R., C.V.G., S.N., E.S. and M.D.L.H.

Funding: This research received no external funding.

Conflicts of Interest: D.R.: Consultant for Fujifilm Sonosite, Consultant for and funded research from General Electric, Medical Advisory Board Member–EchoNous.

References

1. Robinson, M.D.; Branham, A.R.; Locklear, A.; Robertson, S.; Gridley, T. Measuring Satisfaction and Usability of FaceTime for Virtual Visits in Patients with Uncontrolled Diabetes. *Telemed. J. E Health* **2015**. [CrossRef] [PubMed]
2. Wu, X.; Oliveria, S.A.; Yagerman, S.; Chen, L.; DeFazio, J.; Braun, R.; Marghoob, A.A. Feasibility and Efficacy of Patient-Initiated Mobile Teledermoscopy for Short-term Monitoring of Clinically Atypical Nevi. *Jama Derm.* **2015**, *151*, 489–496. [CrossRef] [PubMed]
3. Williams, G.W.; Buendia, F.I.; Idowu, O.O. Utilization of a mobile videoconferencing tool (FaceTime) for real-time evaluation of critically ill neurosurgical patients. *J. Neurosurg. Anesth.* **2015**, *27*, 72. [CrossRef] [PubMed]
4. Miyashita, T.; Iketani, Y.; Nagamine, Y.; Goto, T. FaceTime®for teaching ultrasound-guided anesthetic procedures in remote place. *J. Clin. Monit. Comput* **2014**, *28*, 211–215. [CrossRef] [PubMed]
5. Van Oeveren, L.; Donner, J.; Fantegrossi, A.; Mohr, N.M.; Brown, C.A., 3rd. Telemedicine-Assisted Intubation in Rural Emergency Departments: A National Emergency Airway Registry Study. *Telemed. J. E Health* **2017**, *23*, 290–297. [CrossRef] [PubMed]

6. Moore, C.L.; Copel, J.A. Point-of-care ultrasonography. *N. Engl. J. Med.* **2011**, *364*, 749–757. [CrossRef] [PubMed]
7. P&S Market Reseach. Available online: https://globenewswire.com/news-release/2017/07/21/1055557/0/en/Point-of-Care-Ultrasound-PoCUS-Device-Market-to-Grow-at-6-9-CAGR-till-2025-P-S-Market-Research.html (accessed on 4 February 2019).
8. Wang, S.; Parsons, M.; Stone-McLean, J.; Rogers, P.; Boyd, S.; Hoover, K.; Meruvia-Pastor, O.; Gong, M.; Smith, A. Augmented Reality as a Telemedicine Platform for Remote Procedural Training. *Sensors* **2017**, *17*, 2294. [CrossRef] [PubMed]
9. Levine, A.R.; McCurdy, M.T.; Zubrow, M.T.; Papali, A.; Mallemat, H.A.; Verceles, A.C. Tele-intensivists can instruct non-physicians to acquire high-quality ultrasound images. *J. Crit. Care* **2015**, *30*, 871–875. [CrossRef] [PubMed]
10. Henwood, P.C.; Mackenzie, D.C.; Rempell, J.S.; Douglass, E.; Dukundane, D.; Liteplo, A.S.; Leo, M.M.; Murray, A.F.; Vaillancourt, S.; Dean, A.J.; et al. Intensive point-of-care ultrasound training with long-term follow-up in a cohort of Rwandan physicians. *Trop. Med. Int. Health* **2016**, *21*, 1531–1538. [CrossRef] [PubMed]
11. Choo, E.K.H.; Chen, R.; Millington, S.J.; Hibbert, B.; Tran, D.T.T.; Posner, G.; Sohmer, B. Remote solutions for telementoring point-of-care ultrasound echocardiography: The RESOLUTE study. *Can. J. Anaesth.* **2017**, *64*, 1077–1078. [CrossRef] [PubMed]
12. Smith, A.; Addison, R.; Rogers, P.; Stone-McLean, J.; Boyd, S.; Hoover, K.; Pollard, M.; Dubrowski, A.; Parsons, M. Remote Mentoring of Point-of-Care Ultrasound Skills to Inexperienced Operators Using Multiple Telemedicine Platforms: Is a Cell Phone Good Enough? *J. Ultrasound Med.* **2018**, *37*, 2517–2525. [CrossRef] [PubMed]
13. Kolbe, N.; Killu, K.; Coba, V.; Neri, L.; Garcia, K.M.; McCulloch, M.; Spreafico, A.; Dulchavsky, S. Point of care ultrasound (POCUS) telemedicine project in rural Nicaragua and its impact on patient management. *J. Ultrasound* **2015**, *18*, 179–185. [CrossRef] [PubMed]
14. Robertson, T.E.; Levine, A.R.; Verceles, A.C.; Buchner, J.A.; Lantry, J.H., 3rd; Papali, A.; Zubrow, M.T.; Colas, L.N.; Augustin, M.E.; McCurdy, M.T.; et al. Remote tele-mentored ultrasound for non-physician learners using FaceTime: A feasibility study in a low-income country. *J. Crit. Care* **2017**, *40*, 145–148. [CrossRef] [PubMed]
15. Policy, T.C.f.C.H. Available online: https://www.cchpca.org/sites/default/files/2019-05/cchp_report_MASTER_spring_2019_FINAL.pdf (accessed on 23 October 2019).

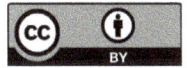

© 2019 by the authors. Licensee MDPI, Basel, Switzerland. This article is an open access article distributed under the terms and conditions of the Creative Commons Attribution (CC BY) license (http://creativecommons.org/licenses/by/4.0/).

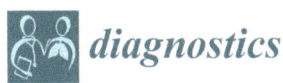

Editorial

Blockchain and Artificial Intelligence Technology for Novel Coronavirus Disease 2019 Self-Testing

Tivani P. Mashamba-Thompson [1,*] and Ellen Debra Crayton [2]

[1] Department of Public Health, University of Limpopo, Polokwane, Limpopo Province 0727, South Africa
[2] Genesis Technology and Management Group, (GenesisTMG, LLC), Bethesda, MD 20817, USA; Ellen.Crayton@genesistmg.com
* Correspondence: tivani.mashamba@ul.ac.za

Received: 26 March 2020; Accepted: 31 March 2020; Published: 1 April 2020

Abstract: The novel coronavirus disease 2019 (COVID-19) is rapidly spreading with a rising death toll and transmission rate reported in high income countries rather than in low income countries. The overburdened healthcare systems and poor disease surveillance systems in resource-limited settings may struggle to cope with this COVID-19 outbreak and this calls for a tailored strategic response for these settings. Here, we recommend a low cost blockchain and artificial intelligence-coupled self-testing and tracking systems for COVID-19 and other emerging infectious diseases. Prompt deployment and appropriate implementation of the proposed system have the potential to curb the transmissions of COVID-19 and the related mortalities, particularly in settings with poor access to laboratory infrastructure.

Keywords: self-testing; novel coronavirus disease-19; blockchain; artificial intelligence

---

The novel coronavirus disease 2019 (COVID-19) has now reached sub-Saharan Africa (SSA) with cases reported in more than 40 SSA countries. SSA health systems are already battling with poor health outcomes and high mortality rates linked to the unique quadruple (HIV, Tuberculosis and non-communicable diseases) burden of disease [1]. In addition, SSA's dense communities, informal settlements and rural and resource-limited settings are at particular risk and are most vulnerable to the COVID-19 outbreak. These populations are underserved in terms of health services and have the potential to become to new COVID-19 epicenters. The global COVID-19 statistics show surprisingly low transmission rates and fewer deaths in resource-limited countries, particularly countries in Sub-Saharan Africa (SSA). While SSA's young population and warm climate may put SSA at an advantage for coping with the COVID-19 outbreak [2], there is growing concern about the impact of COVID-19 co-infections among the people living with other immune-system-weakening conditions such as HIV, TB and diabetes and the struggling health system in resource-limited settings such as SSA countries [3,4].

There is a growing concern about a failure to find and report cases, especially given weak health systems, inadequate surveillance, insufficient laboratory capacity and limited public health infrastructure in African countries [5]. Access to accurate diagnosis, monitoring and reporting of health outbreaks requires a well-resourced healthcare system [6]. Evidence shows that most resource-limited countries lack an effective, rapid surveillance system [7]. These settings also have a limited availability of health technologies for the electronic surveillance of infectious diseases to facilitate the prevention and containment of emerging infectious diseases such as COVID-19 [7]. Universal health coverage, access to high-quality and timely pathology and laboratory medicine (PALM) services is crucially needed to support health-care systems that are tasked with achieving Sustainable Developmental Goals [8]. This calls for the rapid development and deployment of health innovations for accurate diagnosis and electronic surveillance of COVID-19 in underserved populations.

Recent evidence shows that prompt development and deployment of point-of-care (POC) diagnostics for screening in response to the COVID-19 outbreak can help to curb the spread of the disease and to alleviate the burden on the health system [9,10]. The impact of rapid testing on the COVID-19 death rate has been shown in Germany [11]. Emerging health innovations such as blockchain and artificial intelligence (AI) technology can be coupled with POC diagnostics to enable self-testing of patients in isolation as a result of exposure to COVID-19. Blockchain is a digital, public ledger that records online transactions. It involves the digital distribution of ledger and consensus algorithms and eliminates all the threats of intermediaries [12,13]. One of the commonly-known applications of blockchain is the crypto-currency Bitcoin [14], which has been successfully used as an alternative financial sector in emerging economies including countries in SSA [15]. Blockchain technology has shown adaptability in recent years leading to its incorporation in a wide range of applications including biomedical and healthcare systems [16–18]. The use of blockchain and AI in healthcare is evident in the following areas: management of electronic medical records; drugs and pharmaceutical supply chain management; biomedical research; education; remote patient monitoring; and health data analytics [17].

Mobile connected point-of-care diagnostics and self-testing has been successfully implemented in resource-limited settings [19–21]. However, there is limited evidence on the use of blockchain and AI technology for disease diagnosis. Bearing in mind the era of COVID-19 and the evidence on the overburdened healthcare systems and poor disease surveillance systems in resource-limited settings, and taking advantage of the available mobile Health (mHealth) systems, we recommend, a rapid development and deployment of low cost blockchain and AI-coupled mHealth connected self-testing and tracking systems as one of the strategic response strategies for COVID-19 and other immerging infectious diseases (Figure 1).

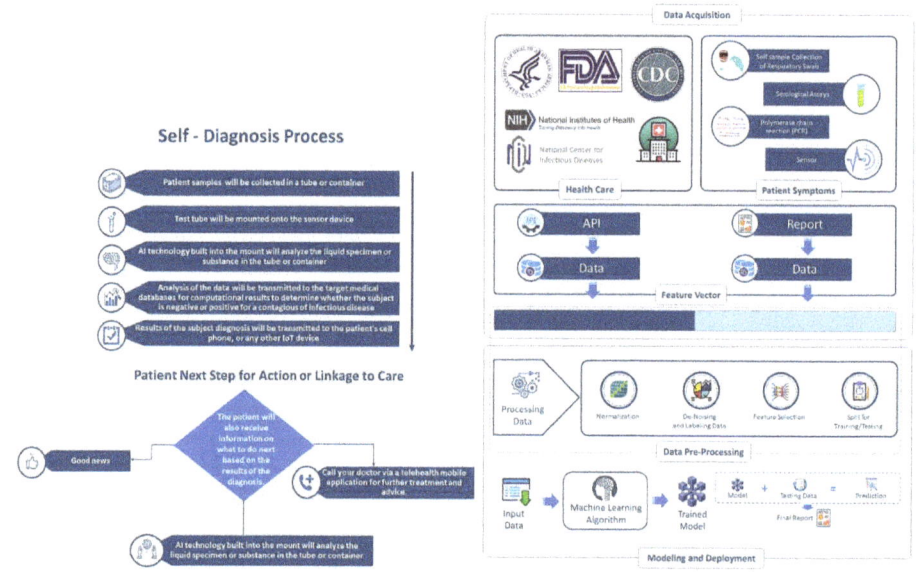

Figure 1. Proposed community-based blockchain and artificial intelligence-coupled mobile-linked self-testing and tracking system for emerging infectious diseases.

The initial step for this system is through a mobile phone or tablet application (app) which could be adapted from existing self-testing apps [22,23]. The app will request a user's personal identifier before opening pre-testing instructions. Following testing, the user will upload results into the app. The blockchain and AI system will enable the transfer of the test result to alert the outbreak surveillance authorities of all tests performed as well as the number of positive and negative test results. This will help ensure that all positive cases are referred to a quarantine site for treatment and monitoring. The in-built geographic information system (GIS) in mobile devices will enable the tracking of the people who tested positive. This system will also be connected to the local and international databases to ensure appropriate surveillance and control of the outbreak.

The AI component of this technology will enable potent power in data collection (patient information, geographic location of the patient and test results), security, analysis, and curation of disparate and clinical data sets from federated blockchain platforms to derive triangulated data at very high degrees of confidence and speed. With this well-architected integrative technology platform, we assure secure and immutable data sets that enable the collection of high-quality data and can draw deep insights. Local development of these diagnostics can help overcome the supply chain challenges [24] and the cost which can limit accessibility of POC diagnostics in resource-limited settings. This technology can be adapted for use in community-based case finding of other infectious diseases such as HIV, TB and Malaria, which may be exacerbated by the current COVID-19 outbreak. Relevant stakeholders' involvement will be crucial to ensure the efficient development and sustainable implementation of the proposed technology, particularly in underserved populations.

Funding: This research received no external funding.

Conflicts of Interest: The authors declare no conflict of interest.

References

1. Institute for Health Metrics and Evaluation (IHME). *Findings from the Global Burden of Disease Study 2017*; IHME: Seattle, WA, USA, 2018; Available online: https://www.healthdata.org/sites/default/files/files/policy_report/2019/GBD_2017_Booklet.pdf (accessed on 25 March 2020).
2. Chopera, D. Can Africa Withstand COVID-19. Available online: https://www.project-syndicate.org/commentary/africa-covid19-advantages-disadvantages-by-denis-chopera-2020-03-2020-03. (accessed on 25 March 2020).
3. Wong, E. TB, HIV and COVID-19: Urgent Questions as Three Epidemics Collide. Available online: https://theconversation.com/tb-hiv-and-covid-19-urgent-questions-as-three-epidemics-collide-134554?fbclid=IwAR3ycjutsVRKxcRjxcsO4Vaw_-yyKf16Gey3GTMeAejvZVsACcf9CgqHP0Q (accessed on 25 March 2020).
4. Loven, C.N. On-Again, Off-Again Looks to Be Best Social-Distancing Option. Available online: https://news.harvard.edu/gazette/story/2020/03/how-to-prevent-overwhelming-hospitals-and-build-immunity/ (accessed on 28 March 2020).
5. Whiteside, A. Covid-19 Watch: The Crisis Deepens. In Covid-19 Watch: The Crisis Deepens. Available online: https://alan-whiteside.com/2020/03/25/covid-19-watch-the-crisis-deepens-2/?fbclid=IwAR3RkSOESoQzkxT4kKsIAYmDOPG9t39qoCUYQxmVLg-tnBmMtB6Zm-FpuTY (accessed on 25 March 2020).
6. Herida, M.; Dervaux, B.; Desenclos, J.-C. Economic evaluations of public health surveillance systems: A systematic review. *Eur. J. Public Health* **2016**, *26*, 674–680. [CrossRef] [PubMed]
7. Rattanaumpawan, P.; Boonyasiri, A.; Vong, S.; Thamlikitkul, V. Systematic review of electronic surveillance of infectious diseases with emphasis on antimicrobial resistance surveillance in resource-limited settings. *Am. J. Infect. Control* **2018**, *46*, 139–146. [CrossRef]
8. United Nations. The Sustainable Development Goals Report 2019. Available online: https://unstats.un.org/sdgs/report/2019/The-Sustainable-Development-Goals-Report-2019.pdf. (accessed on 19 March 2020).
9. Pang, J.; Wang, M.X.; Ang, I.Y.H.; Tan, S.H.X.; Lewis, R.F.; Chen, J.I.-P.; Gutierrez, R.A.; Gwee, S.X.W.; Chua, P.E.Y.; Yang, Q. Potential rapid diagnostics, vaccine and therapeutics for 2019 novel coronavirus (2019-nCoV): A systematic review. *J. Clin. Med.* **2020**, *9*, 623. [CrossRef]
10. Wang, C.; Horby, P.W.; Hayden, F.G.; Gao, G.F. A novel coronavirus outbreak of global health concern. *Lancet* **2020**, *395*, 470–473. [CrossRef]

11. U.S. News. Experts: Rapid Testing Helps Explain Few German Virus Deaths. Available online: https://www.usnews.com/news/health-news/articles/2020-03-09/experts-rapid-testing-helps-explain-few-german-virus-deaths (accessed on 19 March 2020).
12. Yaqoob, S.; Khan, M.; Talib, R.; Butt, A.; Saleem, S.; Arif, F.; Nadeem, A. Use of Blockchain in Healthcare: A Systematic Literature Review. *Int. J. Adv. Comput. Sci. Appl.* **2019**, *10*, 644–653. [CrossRef]
13. Gomez, M.; Bustamante, P.; Weiss, M.B.; Murtazashvili, I.; Madison, M.J.; Law, W.; Mylovanov, T.; Bodon, H.; Krishnamurthy, P. Is Blockchain the Next Step in the Evolution Chain of [Market] Intermediaries? Available online: https://ssrn.com/abstract=3427506 (accessed on 25 March 2020).
14. Nakamoto, S.; Bitcoin, A. A Peer-To-Peer Electronic Cash System. Available online: https://bitcoin.org/bitcoin.pdf (accessed on 25 March 2020).
15. Vincent, O.; Evans, O. Can cryptocurrency, mobile phones, and internet herald sustainable financial sector development in emerging markets? *J. Trans. Manag.* **2019**, *24*, 259–279. [CrossRef]
16. Mettler, M. Blockchain technology in healthcare: The revolution starts here. In Proceedings of the 2016 IEEE 18th international conference on e-health networking, applications and services (Healthcom), Munich, Germany, 14–16 September 2016; pp. 1–3.
17. Agbo, C.C.; Mahmoud, Q.H.; Eklund, J.M. Blockchain technology in healthcare: A systematic review. *Healthcare* **2019**, *7*, 56. [CrossRef] [PubMed]
18. Zhang, P.; Schmidt, D.C.; White, J.; Lenz, G. Blockchain technology use cases in healthcare. In *Advances in Computers*; Elsevier: New York, NY, USA, 2018; Volume 111, pp. 1–41.
19. Makhudu, S.J.; Kuupiel, D.; Gwala, N.; Mashamba-Thompson, T.P. The Use of Patient Self-Testing in Low-and Middle-Income Countries: A Systematic Scoping Review. *Point Care* **2019**, *18*, 9–16. [CrossRef]
20. Bervell, B.; Al-Samarraie, H. A comparative review of mobile health and electronic health utilization in sub-Saharan African countries. *Soc. Sci. Med.* **2019**, *232*, 1–16. [CrossRef] [PubMed]
21. Adeagbo, O.; Kim, H.-Y.; Tanser, F.; Xulu, S.; Dlamini, N.; Gumede, V.; Mathenjwa, T.; Bärnighausen, T.; McGrath, N.; Blandford, A. Acceptability of a tablet-based application to support early HIV testing among men in rural KwaZulu-Natal, South Africa: A mixed method study. *AIDS Care* **2020**, 1–8. [CrossRef] [PubMed]
22. Pai, N.P.; Behlim, T.; Abrahams, L.; Vadnais, C.; Shivkumar, S.; Pillay, S.; Binder, A.; Deli-Houssein, R.; Engel, N.; Joseph, L. Will an unsupervised self-testing strategy for HIV work in health care workers of South Africa? A cross sectional pilot feasibility study. *PLoS ONE* **2013**, *8*, e79772.
23. Tay, I.; Garland, S.; Gorelik, A.; Wark, J.D. Development and testing of a mobile phone app for self-monitoring of calcium intake in young women. *JMIR mHealth and uHealth* **2017**, *5*, e27. [CrossRef] [PubMed]
24. Kuupiel, D.; Bawontuo, V.; Mashamba-Thompson, T.P. Improving the accessibility and efficiency of point-of-care diagnostics Services in low-and Middle-Income Countries: Lean and agile supply chain management. *Diagnostics* **2017**, *7*, 58. [CrossRef] [PubMed]

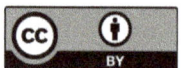

© 2020 by the authors. Licensee MDPI, Basel, Switzerland. This article is an open access article distributed under the terms and conditions of the Creative Commons Attribution (CC BY) license (http://creativecommons.org/licenses/by/4.0/).

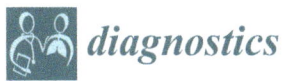

Review

Electronic Health Information Systems to Improve Disease Diagnosis and Management at Point-of-Care in Low and Middle Income Countries: A Narrative Review

Thokozani Khubone [1,*], Boikhutso Tlou [1] and Tivani Phosa Mashamba-Thompson [1,2]

1. Department of Public Health Medicine, School of Nursing and Public Health, University of KwaZulu-Natal, Durban 4041, South Africa; Tlou@ukzn.ac.za (B.T.); Mashamba-Thompson@ukzn.ac.za (T.P.M.-T.)
2. Department of Public Health, Faculaty of Health Sciences, University of Limpopo, Polokwane 0727, South Africa
* Correspondence: khubone.thokozani04@gmail.com

Received: 20 March 2020; Accepted: 7 May 2020; Published: 21 May 2020

Abstract: The purpose of an electronic health information system (EHIS) is to support health care workers in providing health care services to an individual client and to enable data exchange among service providers. The demand to explore the use of EHIS for diagnosis and management of communicable and non-communicable diseases has increased dramatically due to the volume of patient data and the need to retain patients in care. In addition, the advent of Coronavirus disease 2019 (COVID-19) pandemic in high disease burdened low and middle income countries (LMICs) has increased the need for robust EHIS to enable efficient surveillance of the pandemic. EHIS has potential to enable efficient delivery of disease diagnostics services at point-of-care (POC) and reduce medical errors. This review provides an overview of literature on EHIS's with a focus on describing the key components of EHIS and presenting evidence on enablers and barriers to implementation of EHISs in LMICs. With guidance from the presented evidence, we proposed EHIS key stakeholders' roles and responsibilities to ensure efficient utility of EHIS for disease diagnosis and management at POC in LMICs.

Keywords: electronic health information system; diagnosis; treatment; point-of-care; low and middle income countries

1. Introduction

The health sector is lagging behind in the era of information and technology (IT). The main purpose for use of IT in the health sector include the following: extending geographic access to health care; enhancing client communication with the health provider; improving disease diagnosis and treatment; improved data quality management; and to avoid fraud and abuse of client's confidentiality [1–3]. The introduction of digitization has revealed the possibilities and costs benefits to health care management. IT systems such as electronic health information systems (EHIS) have been shown to be a useful tool for improving disease diagnosis and treatment at point of care (POC), globally [4–6]. EHIS is the digital version of a patients' paper chart, which has capacity to store health data such as test results and treatments. It is also designed to enable real-time, patient-centered records that make information available instantly and securely to the authorized users [7]. The term EHIS is used interchangeably with electronic health records (EHRs), eHealth and electronic medical records (EMRs). EHIS are a vital part of health IT built to go beyond standard clinical data collected in a providers' office and can be inclusive of a broader view of a patient care [8].

An efficient functioning EHIS requires the use of digital health systems such as three interlinked electronic register (Tier.Net), which has an ability to facilitate information exchange between software [9]. Tier.Net is used by healthcare facilities to enable electronic collection, storage, management and sharing of patient's electronic health or medical records for the purpose of patient care, research and quality management [10]. Countries are currently battling with a global pandemic caused by the outbreak of SARS COV-2, a virus that causes Coronavirus disease 2019 (COVID-19). The advent of COVID-19 in high disease burdened low and middle income countries (LMICs) such as South Africa has increased the need for robust EHIS to enable efficient surveillance of the pandemic [11]. The main objective of this review is to presents an overview of literature on the characteristics of EHIS and implementation of EHISs for improving disease diagnosis and treatment at point-of-care in the LMICs. We search for literature from the following databases: PubMed and Google Scholar and included relevant literature from LMICs.

2. Characteristic of Electronic Health Information Systems

An efficiently functioning EHIS is key to health service delivery as it promises a number of substantial benefits, including improving the quality of healthcare service delivery, decreased healthcare costs as well as reduce serious unintended consequences [12]. A poorly implemented EHR system can lead to EHR-related errors that jeopardize the integrity of the information in the EHR, leading to errors that endanger patient safety as well as compromise the quality healthcare services [12]. The following key components are required for an efficient functioning EHIS: patient management component; activity component; clinical component; pharmacy component; laboratory component; radiology information system; and billing system (Figure 1) [13]. Table 1 provides a description on the functions of EHR components within the electronic health system and patient care.

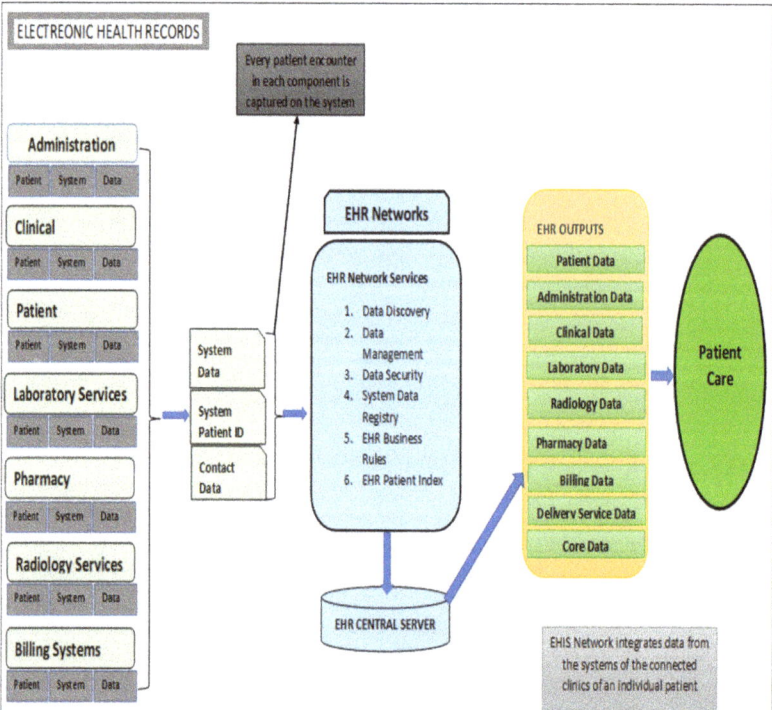

Figure 1. Overview of electronic health information system components (adapted from the National Institute of Health National Center for Reasearch Resources; 2006 [13]).

Table 1. Description of electronic health record (EHR) components, purposes within the electronic health system and patient care by National Institutes of Health National Center for Research Resources.

EHIS Component	Function	Benefit to Patient Care
Patient Management EHIS	Patient registration, admission, transfer and discharge (ADT) functionality. Patient registration includes key patient information such as demographics, insurance information and contact information [14]	Populations and their needs are analyzed at a point of care to determine the services to be rendered to them [15]
Activity EHIS	Flow processed from when a client is entering the point of service till data is digitized on the system [15,16]	Traceability of health data
Clinical EHIS	Habitation of multiple sub-components, e.g., computerized provide order entry (CPOE), electronic documentation, nursing component [14]	Electronic clinical documentation systems enhance the value of EHRs by providing electronic capture of clinical notes; patient assessments; and clinical reports, such as medication administration records (MAR) [13]
Pharmacy EHIS	Islands of automation, such as pharmacy robots for filling prescriptions or payer formularies, that typically are not integrated with EHRs [13]	Improve efficiency of pharmacy services
Laboratory EHIS	Consists of two subcomponents: capturing results from lab machines; and integration with orders, billing and lab machines. The lab component may either be integrated with the EHR or exist as a standalone product [14,17]	Improve efficiency of pathology laboratory services
Radiology Information System and Picture Archiving & Communications System (PACS)	Manages patient workflow, ordering process and results [14]	Enables improved service delivery
The billing system (hospital and professional billing)	Captures all charges generated in the process of taking care of patients. These charges generate claims, which are subsequently submitted to insurance companies, tracked and completed [14]	Tracking of patient data and quality assurance

3. Opportunities Presented by EHIS in the LMICs

Evidence on EHIS in developing countries revealed the following eHealth attributes: tracking of patients who were initiated on treatment; monitoring of adherence to care and early detection of potential loss to follow up; minimize the time it takes to communicate data between different levels; reduction of errors especially the laboratory data; linkage to bar code for unique identification and laboratory samples and the prescription of medication [18]. In Mozambique, a robust electronic patient management system facilitated a facility-level reporting of required indicators, improved ability to identify patients lost to follow-up; and support facility and patient management for HIV care [19]. An implementation study aimed at implementing an integrated pharmaceutical management information system for antiretroviral treatment (ART) and other medicines in Namibia showed the system's reliability in managing ART patients, monitoring ART adherence and HIV drug resistance early warning indicators [20].

4. Enablers of EHIS Implementation in the LMICs

Enables of EHIS implementation in the LMICs are aligned with leadership abilities, sound policy decision and financial support with the goals of purchasing IT, connectivity and capacity building [21]. Enablers for EHIS in LMICs includes: legislation, financial investment; staff training, political leadership; acceptability of technology; performance expectancy; and social influence among professionals [22–24].

4.1. Financial Investment

Many LMICs are supporting financial investment to help scaling up of EHIS. A study from China recommended that in order to achieve the national childhood immunization information management system objectives for 2010, the funding for system-building should be increased [22]. A three-country qualitative study was conducted in southern Africa on the sustainability of health information systems which revealed; more government commitment in funding EHIS such as printer ink, IT infrastructure, recruitment of personnel and running costs [23]. In Ghana, cooperation between the vendors and management was demonstrated [25]. This successful cooperation translated into regularly provision of feedback and sucessful system maintenance [25]. This has helped the facility in alleviating the common challenge faced by most Information Communication and Technology (ICT) implementers in LIMCs [25].

4.2. Legislation

South Africa National Health Act of 2003 is a good example of a legislation, policy, norms and standards defining the role of national, provincial and local governments in terms of EHIS implementation in LMICs [26]. South Africa has advocated the scale up of digital health technologies to improve access to health care and for health systems strengtherning through systems such as Tier.net and District Health Information Software (DHIS and patient registration systems [27]. The delivery of EHIS or eHealth in South Africa's public sector facilities is the responsibility of the provincial departments of health, while policy development resides with the National Department of Health (NDoH). In terms of Section 74 of the National Health Act, the NDoH is also responsible for facilitation and coordination of health information.

4.3. Staff Training

There is growing evidence on the value of well-trained health informatics workforce in LMICs [24]. Studies conducted in Botswana and Uganda showed the on-the-job training and mentorship as a major enabler for EHIS in LMICs [28,29]. This were shown to be an effective approach for strengthening monitoring and evaluation capacity and ensuring data quality within a national health system [28]. It was demonstrated that on-the-job training can also improves performance through timely and increased reporting of key health indicators [29].

4.4. Political Leadership

Effective leadership can positively contribute to the successful adoption of new EHIS in any organization [30]. In Ethiopia, the role of ICT towards universal health coverage prompted academic and political spheres to make ICT on the agenda especially for disease diagnosis and treatment in the LMICs [31]. The Rwandan government has also shown commitment to telemedicine, through their strategic choice of using low-cost and less complex technologies, and strategic partnerships with educational and technology companies to help in the implementation of telemedicine [32].

4.5. Acceptability of Technology

Research has shown that factors such as English language proficiency level, computer literacy and EMR literacy level and education level can influence the level of use of EHIS [33]. Liu and others revealed that the usage of EHIS by health workers in LMICs can be influenced by the level of system simplicity and user friendliness [34]. An economical mobile health application to improve communication between healthcare workers was introduced in KwaZulu-Natal, South Africa using an iterative design process [35]. This application was received positive feedback from healthcare workers due to its ability to improve team spirit between community and clinic based staff [35].

5. Barriers and Challenges to Implemention of EHIS in the LMICs

There are various factors impeding the successful implementation and scale up of EHIS in LMICs. These include the following: complexity of the intervention and lack of technical consensus; limited human resource, poor leadership, insufficient finances, staff resistance, lack of management, low organizational capability; misapplication of proven diffusion techniques; non engagement of both local users and inadequate use of research findings when implementing [36].

5.1. Complexity of the Intervention and Lack of Technical Consensus

The complexity of the EHIS which and lack of consultation as key barriers on the implementation in LMICs [36]. Designing an organizational EHIS with a complex design is a serious threat of the implementation in LMICs [37]. In Rwanda, the interfaces between the existing and new EHIS are the inhibitors to the implementation [38]. There are instances of patient information that are captured into the computer; but challenged with bandwidth requirements in health facilities [39].

5.2. Limited Human Resource

The main barriers in implementing EHIS on the LMICs relate to lack of capacity: human, leadership and management [36]. Human resource capacity is the main barrier not only in terms of the supply but also in terms of the ability to perform the task. The exodus of skilled cadres to the well-paying non-government organizations are the contributing factors to human resource capacity [40].

5.3. Lack of Management

Ineffective coordination, poor management and lack of supervision for EHIS are the main challenges in the LMICs [41,42]. Management capacity and the ability to use data were reported as the root causes in facilities with inadequate human resource, computers and data capturing skills [43]. Late submission of health data and absence of feedback from the supervisors are the key barriers to EHIS implementation in LMICs [44].

5.4. Lack of Funds

EHIS implementation is costly as there is hardware, software, maintenance, training and human resource investment making implementation unaffordable to many LMICs [45]. Cost is the main constraint to adoption and implementation of EHIS in LMICs [46]. Running costs and political will are the prerequisite for sustaining EHIS [40]. Unreliable electricity supply, shortage of IT equipment, poor connectivity and safe accommodation for the equipment are the restraining elements to the successful implementation of EHIS [45].

5.5. Inadequate Health Systems Capacity

Poor public healthcare system with ever changing policies are a hindrances to the successful implementation of the EHIS in LMICs [21]. Leon and others used a framework for assessing the health system challenges to scaling up m-Health in South Africa and revealed a weak ICT environment and limited implementation capacity within the health system [47]. Katuu explored the barriers in improving South African public health sector through eHealth strategy particularly by integrating electronic document and records management system. Inequality, historical red tape and curative structure are the main barriers [48].

5.6. Poor Application of Proven Diffusion Techniques

In Asia, incapacitated human resources and shortage of IT skills were identified as inhibiting factors to EHIS implementation [49]. In Iran, lack of users' knowledge about system and working with it were the barriers identified [50]. In most of the LMICs; the need for a trained workforce in health informatics is great [51]. There are instances where computer illiterate and low morale to use the system are affecting the implementation [36,52]. Some of the challenges include related to EHIS software, cost drivers, interoperability, connectivity in rural set up and data quality [40].

5.7. Staff Resistance

A study conducted in South Africa, demonstrated difficulties with implementing a dual EHIS as a result of clinicians' resistance to using the EHIS and feel more comfortable using paper based system [52]. In Iran, the negative staff attitudes of system developers and lack of acceptability are the main barriers to successful implementation of hospital-based EHIS [50]. Although South Africa EHIS catered for all required information, the hospital officials show poor due to the attitude and resistance to using EHIS for patient treatment and prescriptions [53]. An assessment was conducted by Khasi EHIS state of readiness for rural South African areas, which revealed that the resistance to change and negative perceptions were two key causes for not accepting the intervention. Any new EHIS intervention must address them in order to succeed [54].

5.8. Compromised Data Quality

Studies revealed incompleteness of TB data across multiple information systems in South Africa. Variances between 12% and 38% of the missed cases due to poor recording from the source documents (either patient records or laboratory records) were demonstrated [49,50]. Data collected and reported in the public health system across three large, high HIV-prevalence districts was neither complete nor accurate enough to guide patient tracking as part of prevention of mother to child transmission (PMTCT) care [51].

6. Discussion

This review has provided us with a great platform to depict opportunities of EHIS implementation in LMICs. It has also enabled us to identify and classify barriers and challenges implementation of EHIS that must be addressed pre-implementation to ensure the success. Key to the success of EHIS is the leader's willingness to play a leading role in adopting data demand and supply principles for decision making. The presented literature reveals the need for well-defined roles of EHIS stakeholders to ensure successful implementation and utility. Here, we proposed key stakeholders roles and responsibilities in the implementation of EHIS for disease diagnosis and management at point-of-care (POC) in LMICs (Figure 2). In the proposed key stakeholders' roles and responsibilities we emphasise on that the information culture should be cascaded through different hierarchy levels of an organization. In the absence of the such culture there is likely to be poor adoption, poor data quality and utilization [55].

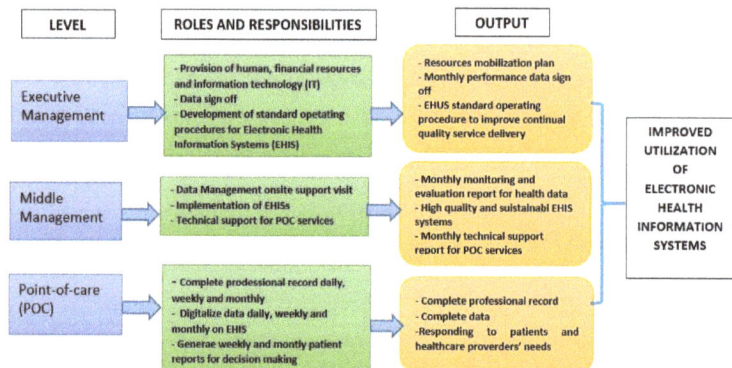

Figure 2. Proposed roles and responsibilities of stakeholders to ensure efficient utility of electronic health information systems for disease diagnosis and treatment at point-of-care in low and middle income counties.

7. Conclusions

The advent of EHIS has revolutionize patient care through improving both disease diagnosis and treatment at POC. However, its use in LMICs is still limited, despite the high disease burden in these settings. EHIS implementation need to be one of the global health priorities to help respond to community's health needs, particularly during the current Covid-19 pandemic. Successful implementation of EHIS requires commitment from health leaders to play a strategic role in terms of the policy directive, resource mobilization and evidence-based decision-making. To help optimize the implementation and use of EHIS in LMICs, we have proposed roles and responsibilities of stakeholders to ensure efficient and sustainable implementation of EHIS. A systematic approach for stakeholder engagement would be crucial to ensuring successful operationalization of the proposed roles and responsibilities.

Author Contributions: T.K., T.P.M.-T., B.T. conceptualized the study. T.K. produced the first draft of the manuscript. T.P.M.-T. and B.T. commented on this draft and contributed to the final version. All authors have read and agreed to the published version of the manuscript.

Funding: This research received no external funding.

Acknowledgments: We would like to thank the KwaZulu-Natal Department of Health for granting us access to library databases and referencing software.

Conflicts of Interest: The authors declare no conflicts of interest.

References

1. Makanga, P.T.; Schuurman, N.; von Dadelszen, P.; Firoz, T. A scoping review of geographic information systems in maternal health. *Int. J. Gynaecol. Obstet.* **2016**, *134*, 13–17. [CrossRef]
2. Kyriacou, E.; Pavlopoulos, S.; Berler, A.; Neophytou, M.; Bourka, A.; Georgoulas, A.; Anagnostaki, A.; Karayiannis, D.; Schizas, C.; Pattichis, C.; et al. Multi-purpose HealthCare Telemedicine Systems with mobile communication link support. *Biomed. Eng. Online* **2003**, *2*, 7. [CrossRef] [PubMed]
3. Cohen, G.; Goldsmith, J.; Roller, P.S.; Widran, S.; Patterson, G.W.; Daugherty, J.R.; Van Antwerp, W.P. Medical Data Management System and Process. U.S. Patent 8, 313.433 B2, 20 November 2012.
4. Muller-Staub, M. *Evaluation of the Implementation of Nursing Diagnostics. A Study of the Use of Nursing Diagnoses, Interventions and Outcomes in Nursing Documentation*; Blackwell Publishing LTD: Oxford, UK, 2007.
5. Müller-Staub, M. Evaluation of the implementation of nursing diagnoses, interventions, and outcomes. *Int. J. Nurs. Terminol. Classif.* **2009**, *20*, 9–15. [CrossRef] [PubMed]
6. Hunt, D.L.; Haynes, R.B.; Hanna, S.E.; Smith, K.J.J. Effects of computer-based clinical decision support systems on physician performance and patient outcomes: A systematic review. *JAMA* **1998**, *280*, 1339–1346. [CrossRef] [PubMed]
7. Brook, C. What is a Health Information System? Available online: https://digitalguardian.com/blog/what-health-information-system (accessed on 15 May 2020).
8. HealthIT.Gov. What is an electronic health record (EHR)? National Coordinator for Health Information Technology 2018. Available online: https://www.healthit.gov/faq/what-electronic-health-record-ehr (accessed on 15 May 2020).
9. Osler, M.; Hilderbrand, K.; Hennessey, C.; Arendse, J.; Goemaere, E.; Ford, N.; Boulle, A. A three-tier framework for monitoring antiretroviral therapy in high HIV burden settings. *J. Int. Aids Soc.* **2014**, *17*, 18908. [CrossRef] [PubMed]
10. Elgujja, A.A. Impact of Information Technology on Patient Confidentiality Rights: A Perspectives. In *Impacts of Information Technology on Patient Care and Empowerment*; IGI Global: Hershey, PA, USA, 2020.
11. Mashamba-Thompson, T.P.; Crayton, E.D. Blockchain and Artificial Intelligence Technology for Novel Coronavirus Disease-19 Self-Testing. *Diagnostics* **2020**, *10*, 198. [CrossRef] [PubMed]
12. Bowman, S. Impact of electronic health record systems on information integrity: Quality and safety implications. *Perspect. Health Inf. Manag.* **2013**, *10*, 1c. [PubMed]
13. National Institutes of Health. Electronic health records overview. In *National Center for Research Resources*; National Institutes of Health: Bethesda, MD, USA, 2006.

14. Basic Components of Electronic Health Record. Available online: https://rxvisor.com/2013/12/28/2013-12-28-basic-components-of-an-electronic-health-record/ (accessed on 15 May 2020).
15. Hartzler, A.; McCarty, C.A.; Rasmussen, L.V.; Williams, M.S.; Brilliant, M.; Bowton, E.A.; Clayton, E.W.; Faucett, W.A.; Ferryman, K.; Field, J.R.; et al. Stakeholder engagement: A key component of integrating genomic information into electronic health records. *Genet. Med.* **2013**, *15*, 792. [CrossRef]
16. Van de Velde, R.; Degoulet, P. *Clinical Information Systems: A Component-Based Approach*; Springer Science & Business Media: Berlin, Germany, 2003.
17. UKEssays. General Components of an EHR System. Available online: https://www.ukessays.com/essays/information-technology/key-components-of-electronic-health-records-information-technology-essay.php?vref=1 (accessed on 15 May 2020).
18. Blaya, J.A.; Fraser, H.S.; Holt, B. E-health technologies show promise in developing countries. *Health Aff. (Millwood)* **2010**, *29*, 244–251. [CrossRef]
19. Hochgesang, M.; Zamudio-Haas, S.; Moran, L.; Nhampossa, L.; Packel, L.; Leslie, H.; Richard, J.; Shade, S.B. Scaling-up health information systems to improve HIV treatment: An assessment of initial patient monitoring systems in Mozambique. International journal of medical informatics. *Int. J. Med. Inform.* **2017**, *97*, 322–330. [CrossRef]
20. Mabirizi, D.; Phulu, B.; Churfo, W.; Mwinga, S.; Mazibuko, G.; Sagwa, E.; Indongo, L.; Hafner, T. Implementing an Integrated Pharmaceutical Management Information System for Antiretrovirals and Other Medicines: Lessons From Namibia. *Glob. Health Sci. Pract.* **2018**, *6*, 723–735. [CrossRef] [PubMed]
21. Akhlaq, A.; McKinstry, B.; Muhammad, K.B.; Sheikh, A. Barriers and facilitators to health information exchange in low-and middle-income country settings: A systematic review. *Health Policy Plan.* **2016**, *31*, 1310–1325. [CrossRef] [PubMed]
22. Cao, L.-S.; Liu, D.-W.; Guo, B. Progress of childhood immunization information management system in China in 2008. *Zhongguo Yi Miao He Mian Yi* **2009**, *15*, 367–370.
23. Moucheraud, C.; Schwitters, A.; Boudreaux, C.; Giles, D.; Kilmarx, P.H.; Ntolo, N.; Bangani, Z.; St. Louis, M.E.; Bossert, T.J. Sustainability of health information systems: A three-country qualitative study in southern Africa. BMC health services research. *BMC Health Serv. Res.* **2017**, *17*, 23. [CrossRef] [PubMed]
24. Hersh, W. Health and biomedical informatics: Opportunities and challenges for a twenty-first century profession and its education. *Yearb Med. Inform.* **2008**, *17*, 157–164. [CrossRef]
25. Acquah-Swanzy, M. Evaluating Electronic Health Record Systems in Ghana: The Case of Effia Nkwanta Regional Hospital. Master's thesis, UiT Norges Arktiske Universitet, Tromsø, Norway, 2015.
26. National Health Act 61 of 2003. Available online: https://www.gov.za/documents/national-health-act (accessed on 15 May 2020).
27. *National Digital Health Strategy for South Africa 2019–2024*; The National Department of Health Republic of South Africa: Pretoria, South Africa, 2019.
28. Ledikwe, J.H.; Reason, L.L.; Burnett, S.M.; Busang, L.; Bodika, S.; Lebelonyane, R.; Ludick, S.; Matshediso, E.; Mawandia, S.; Mmelesi, M.; et al. Establishing a health information workforce: Innovation for low-and middle-income countries. *Hum. Resour. Health* **2013**, *11*, 35. [CrossRef] [PubMed]
29. Wandera, S.O.; Kwagala, B.; Nankinga, O.; Ndugga, P.; Kabagenyi, A.; Adamou, B.; Kachero, B. Facilitators, best practices and barriers to integrating family planning data in Uganda's health management information system. *BMC Health Serv. Res.* **2019**, *19*, 327. [CrossRef]
30. Ingebrigtsen, T.; Georgiou, A.; Clay-Williams, R.; Magrabi, F.; Hordern, A.; Prgomet, M.; Li, J.; Westbrook, J.; Braithwaite, J. The impact of clinical leadership on health information technology adoption: Systematic review. *Int. J. Med. Inform.* **2014**, *83*, 393–405. [CrossRef]
31. Shiferaw, F.; Zolfo, M. The role of information communication technology (ICT) towards universal health coverage: The first steps of a telemedicine project in Ethiopia. *Glob. Health Action* **2012**, *5*, 1–8.
32. Nchise, A.; Boateng, R.; Mbarika, V.; Saiba, E.; Johnson, O. The challenge of taking baby steps—Preliminary insights into telemedicine adoption in Rwanda. *Health Policy Technol.* **2012**, *1*, 207–213. [CrossRef]
33. Hasanain, R.A.; Vallmuur, K.; Clark, M. Electronic medical record systems in Saudi Arabia: Knowledge and preferences of healthcare professionals. *J. Health Inf. Dev. Ctries.* **2015**, *9*, 1.
34. Liu, C.-F.; Cheng, T.-J. Exploring critical factors influencing physicians' acceptance of mobile electronic medical records based on the dual-factor model: A validation in Taiwan. *BMC Med. Inf. Decis. Mak.* **2015**, *15*, 4.

35. Chaiyachati, K.H.; Loveday, M.; Lorenz, S.; Lesh, N.; Larkan, L.-M.; Cinti, S.; Friedland, G.H.; Haberer, J.E. A pilot study of an mHealth application for healthcare workers: Poor uptake despite high reported acceptability at a rural South African community-based MDR-TB treatment program. *PLoS ONE* **2013**, *8*, e64662. [CrossRef]
36. Yamey, G. What are the barriers to scaling up health interventions in low and middle income countries? A qualitative study of academic leaders in implementation science. *Glob. Health* **2012**, *8*, 11. [CrossRef] [PubMed]
37. Mudaly, T.; Moodley, D.; Pillay, A.; Seebregts, C.J. Architectural Frameworks for Developing National Health Information Systems in Low and Middle Income Countries. In Proceedings of the First International Conference on Enterprise Systems: ES 2013 IEEE, Cape Town, South Africa, 7–8 November 2013.
38. Crichton, R.; Moodley, D.; Pillay, A.; Gakuba, R.; Seebregts, C.J. An architecture and reference implementation of an open health information mediator: Enabling interoperability in the Rwandan health information exchange. In Proceedings of the International Symposium on Foundations of Health Informatics Engineering and Systems, Paris, France, 27–28 August 2012.
39. Ramesh, K.; Shaikh, B.T.; Chandio, A.K.; Jamil, A. Role of Health Management Information System in disease reporting at a rural district of Sindh. *Pak. J. Health* **2012**, *2*, 10–12.
40. Botha, M.; Botha, A.; Herselman, M. The Benefits and Challenges of e-Health Applications: A Content Analysis of the South African Context. In Proceedings of the International Conference on Computer Science, Computer Engineering, and Social Media, Thessaloniki, Greece, 12–14 December 2014.
41. Asangansi, I.; Macleod, B.; Meremikwu, M.; Arikpo, I.; Roberge, D.; Hartsock, B.; Ekinya, I. Improving the routine HMIS in Nigeria through mobile technology for community data collection. *J. Health Inf. Dev. Ctries.* **2013**, *7*, 1.
42. Qazi, M.S.; Ali, M. Pakistan's health management information system: Health managers' perspectives. *J. Pak. Med. Assoc.* **2009**, *59*, 10.
43. Mishra, A.; Vasisht, I.; Kauser, A.; Thiagarajan, S.; Mairembam, D.S. Determinants of Health Management Information Systems performance: Lessons from a district level assessment. *BMC Proc.* **2012**, *6*, 17. [CrossRef]
44. Kapadia-Kundu, N.; Sullivan, T.M.; Safi, B.; Trivedi, G.; Velu, S. Understanding health information needs and gaps in the health care system in Uttar Pradesh, India. *J. Health Commun.* **2012**, *17* (Suppl. 2), 30–45. [CrossRef]
45. Oluoch, T.; de Keizer, N.F. Evaluation of Health IT in Low-Income Countries. *Stud. Health Technol. Inform.* **2016**, *222*, 324–335.
46. Ghia, C.J.; Patil, A.S.; Ved, J.K.; Jha, R. Benefits of telemedicine and barriers to its effective implementation in rural India: A multicentric E-survey. *Indian Med. Gaz.* **2013**, *146*, 1–7.
47. Leon, N.; Schneider, H.; Daviaud, E. Applying a framework for assessing the health system challenges to scaling up mHealth in South Africa. *BMC Med. Inform. Decis. Mak.* **2012**, *12*, 123. [CrossRef]
48. Katuu, S.; Management, T.P. Transforming South Africa's health sector: The eHealth Strategy, the implementation of electronic document and records management systems (EDRMS) and the utility of maturity models. *J. Sci. Technol. Policy Manag.* **2016**, *7*, 330–345. [CrossRef]
49. Dornan, L.; Pinyopornpanish, K.; Jiraporncharoen, W.; Hashmi, A.; Dejkriengkraikul, N.; Angkurawaranon, C. Utilisation of Electronic Health Records for Public Health in Asia: A Review of Success Factors and Potential Challenges. *BioMed Res. Int.* **2019**, *2019*, 7341841. [CrossRef] [PubMed]
50. Ahmadian, L.; Khajouei, R.; Nejad, S.S.; Ebrahimzadeh, M.; Nikkar, S. Prioritizing barriers to successful implementation of hospital information systems. *J. Med. Syst.* **2014**, *38*, 151. [CrossRef]
51. Luna, D.; Almerares, A.; Mayan, J.C.; Gonzalez Bernaldo de Quiros, F.; Otero, C. Health informatics in developing countries: Going beyond pilot practices to sustainable implementations: A review of the current challenges. *Healthc Inform Res.* **2014**, *20*, 3–10. [CrossRef]
52. Ohuabunwa, E.C.; Sun, J.; Jubanyik, K.J.; Wallis, L. Electronic Medical Records in low to middle income countries: The case of Khayelitsha Hospital, South Africa. *Afr. J. Emerg. Med.* **2016**, *6*, 38–43. [CrossRef]
53. Marutha, N.S.; Ngulube, P. Electronic records management in the public health sector of the Limpopo province in South Africa. *Inform. Dev.* **2012**, *45*, 39–67.

54. Kgasi, M.; Kalema, B. Assessment E-health readiness for rural South African areas. *J. Ind. Intell. Inf.* **2014**, *2*, 2. [CrossRef]
55. Skiti, V. Qualitative Assessment of the Utilisation of Tier.Net Health Information among facility and programme managers In Ekurhuleni district, Gauteng. Available online: http://hdl.handle.net/11394/5942 (accessed on 15 May 2020).

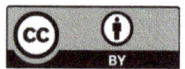

© 2020 by the authors. Licensee MDPI, Basel, Switzerland. This article is an open access article distributed under the terms and conditions of the Creative Commons Attribution (CC BY) license (http://creativecommons.org/licenses/by/4.0/).

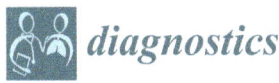

Article

Improving Access to Diagnostics for Schistosomiasis Case Management in Oyo State, Nigeria: Barriers and Opportunities

G-Young Van [1], Adeola Onasanya [1], Jo van Engelen [1,2], Oladimeji Oladepo [3] and Jan Carel Diehl [1,*]

[1] Sustainable Design Engineering, Delft University of Technology, 2628CE Delft, The Netherlands; g.y.van@tudelft.nl (G.-Y.V.); A.A.Onasanya@tudelft.nl (A.O.); J.M.L.vanEngelen@tudelft.nl (J.v.E.)
[2] Department of Economics and Business, University of Groningen, 9747AE Groningen, The Netherlands
[3] Department of Health Promotion and Education, University of Ibadan, 200212 Ibadan, Nigeria; oladepod@yahoo.com
* Correspondence: j.c.diehl@tudelft.nl; Tel.: +31-614-015-469

Received: 4 May 2020; Accepted: 18 May 2020; Published: 20 May 2020

Abstract: Schistosomiasis is one of the Neglected Tropical Diseases that affects over 200 million people worldwide, of which 29 million people in Nigeria. The principal strategy for schistosomiasis in Nigeria is a control and elimination program which comprises a school-based Mass Drug Administration (MDA) with limitations of high re-infection rates and the exclusion of high-risk populations. The World Health Organization (WHO) recommends guided case management of schistosomiasis (diagnostic tests or symptom-based detection plus treatment) at the Primary Health Care (PHC) level to ensure more comprehensive morbidity control. However, these require experienced personnel with sufficient knowledge of symptoms and functioning laboratory equipment. Little is known about where, by whom and how diagnosis is performed at health facilities within the case management of schistosomiasis in Nigeria. Furthermore, there is a paucity of information on patients' health-seeking behaviour from the onset of disease symptoms until a cure is obtained. In this study, we describe both perspectives in Oyo state, Nigeria and address the barriers using adapted health-seeking stages and access framework. The opportunities for improving case management were identified, such as a prevalence study of high-risk groups, community education and screening, enhancing diagnostic capacity at the PHC through point-of-care diagnostics and strengthening the capability of health workers.

Keywords: schistosomiasis; barriers to diagnostics; access to healthcare; end-user perspectives; neglected tropical diseases; Nigeria; case management

1. Introduction

Schistosomiasis is a parasitic disease that affects over 200 million people around the world, and 90% of the infected population are in African countries. These countries have the highest burden of morbidity and mortality [1]. Nigeria is the most endemic country in Sub-Saharan Africa with 101.3 million people at risk, and 29 million infected [2]. The infection can cause anaemia, growth stunting, cognitive impairment, decreased productivity and long-term health consequences such as bladder cancer and infertility [3]. Despite its high socio-economic burden [4], it has received limited attention from governments and stakeholders in healthcare settings, similarly to other Neglected Tropical Disease [2]. Although a prevalence study for schistosomiasis in Nigeria was conducted in 2015 [5], the selection of the sample collection was limited to children and did not address other high-risk groups such as adults [6,7].

Currently, vertical and horizontal programs are used for schistosomiasis control in Nigeria [8]. The control and elimination program is a vertical approach and a principal strategy for control of schistosomiasis (and other NTDs). The horizontal approach is the case management of individual cases at the primary health care level [9]. The control and elimination program provides annual mass treatment of praziquantel for school-age children aged 5 to 14, who are known as the most heavily infected part of the population [10]. Praziquantel has been reported to be a safe and effective treatment, and this approach is said to significantly reduce the prevalence of schistosomiasis and the intensity of infection in high endemic areas [11]. However, three major limitations characterised this approach including high re-infection rates [12], unsustainable mapping and delivery with its high dependency on donations of praziquantel [13,14], and exclusion of other high-risk groups such as people who frequently have contact with water for domestic and professional purposes [2,11].

In light of these limitations, there is a need to pay more attention to the horizontal approach (case management) because it can provide more sustainable, efficient and more localized interventions [9]. The case management approach, which is strongly recommended by the WHO, focuses on diagnosis and treatment [15,16]. In the event that the health facility does not have the diagnostic capability, symptom-based case detection is recommended. This approach has strong potentials in reducing disease transmission by shortening the infectious period of patients through early diagnosis and immediate treatment which will result in improved treatment outcomes [16].

The standard method for schistosomiasis diagnosis is microscopic examination in a lab-setting. The samples for *Schistosoma haematobium* (*S. haematobium*) are prepared either by urine filtration (using polycarbonate filters) or centrifugation. The samples for *Schistosoma mansoni* (*S. mansoni*) are prepared by Kato Katz faecal smear [17,18]. The challenges for sample preparation within sub-Saharan African context include the shortage of lab technicians and equipment at primary health care level [19] as well as the high labour-intensiveness and initial and maintenance costs [18]. There are alternative diagnostics methods, however, they have limitations [17]. Methods such as questionnaires, visible haematuria and urine reagent strips are available but have low sensitivity and specificity. Antibody or antigen detection-based tests are not yet commercially available. Point-of-care circulating cathodic antigen (CCA) test is on the market with high sensitivity and specificity, yet it is more specific to *S. mansoni* and has a disadvantage in affordability. For the health facilities without diagnostic capability, the WHO suggests the symptom-based case detection and treatment [15,16]. This is, for example currently being used in Ghana where the healthcare workers relate blood in urine (hematuria, dysuria) to *S. haematobium* and blood in stool and abdominal discomfort to *S. mansoni* [20]. Although the symptom-based case detection seems to be an effective method for morbidity control in high endemic areas with low resources, the detection depends on the knowledge of the health workers and prior-experience with schistosomiasis patients. There is a high possibility of failing to suspect cases with non-distinct symptoms [20,21]. It is also not clear if praziquantel is available at all levels of the healthcare system to treat the confirmed cases.

Overall, having an adequate diagnostic capability is essential to proper case management, but this requires skilled personnel with sufficient knowledge and functioning equipment. There have been reports indicating poor availability of basic equipment at the primary health care facilities in Nigeria and questions have also been raised about the quality of service delivery [22,23]. This can affect the diagnostic capability within the context of case management of schistosomiasis control. Nonetheless, to our knowledge, there is no specific study that has explored this aspect critically.

Apart from the diagnostic capabilities within the healthcare system, the disease awareness and knowledge of patients can affect health-seeking behaviour. Case management works with passive case detection, which is usually triggered by patients taking action to seek care based on a number of factors. A study in Kano state in Nigeria [24] indicates that the majority of the study participants did not have knowledge on cause, signs, and symptoms of schistosomiasis, even though the majority of them indicated that they are aware of the disease. In addition, only 35% indicated that they would seek treatment from clinics and hospitals. Another study in Adamawa state in Nigeria [25] showed that around 40% of its study participants did not seek any care, 30% visited the patent medicine vendor, while only 17% went to the hospitals. It is of note that patients, when seeking care, have a high preference toward self-medication or use of traditional healers, which may be due to the poverty and physical inaccessibility [24,25]. Nevertheless, there are information gaps on whether and how the patients become aware of the early signs after getting infected, and what barriers prevent them from taking action to seek care.

Therefore, the objective of this research is to explore how the case management currently takes place in Nigeria and to identify the barriers to access from patients and healthcare workers perspective by using empirical data. This would assist us in making appropriate recommendations for future improvement on the case management.

2. Materials and Methods

This study was conducted as part of the interdisciplinary research project "INSPiRED"—Inclusive diagnoStics For Poverty RElated parasitic Diseases in Nigeria and Gabon funded by NWO—WOTRO Science for Global Development programme. The INSPiRED project aims to design and deliver new technical interventions for diagnostics of malaria, schistosomiasis and hookworm infection in close co-creation with local stakeholders.

2.1. Ethics

The study protocol was approved by the UI/UCH Joint Ethical Review Committee of University of Ibadan (10 Dec 2019) and with registration number NHREC/05/01/2008a. Study participants were provided with an information sheet explaining the objectives of the study, and all participants signed or verbally agreed to informed consent forms prior to participation.

2.2. Study Setting

This study took place in Oyo State, one of the 36 states in Nigeria, with an estimated population of 7.8 million people [26]. Data for this study were collected in December 2019 from two Local Government Areas (LGAs) of Oyo State; Ibadan North and Akinyele which are based in urban and rural areas respectively. The selection was based on their moderate-to-high prevalence of schistosomiasis and accessibility to the interviewees.

2.3. Study Sample

The study sample consisted of five categories of stakeholder based on a literature review and expert suggestions (See Table 1). All 29 respondents were purposively selected. They were contacted and informed about the research by the local research coordinator prior to the study.

Table 1. Stakeholder categories and respondents.

	Stakeholder Categories	Respondents	LGA
1	Community members who have experience with schistosomiasis	6 Parents/Guardians of people who were treated for schistosomiasis	Ibadan North, Akinyele
2	Stakeholders within community that can impact on the patient decision to access care	1 Traditional healer 1 Community leader 1 Patent Medicine Vendor (PMV)	[1] Ibadan North
3	Stakeholders in the formal health care	2 Community Health worker 2 Community mobilizers 1 Doctor 5 Lab personnel	Ibadan North, Akinyele
4	Stakeholders within Local and State Government	1 Medical Officer of Health/PHC Coordinator 2 Disease Surveillance Notification Officers (DSNO) 1 PHC Coordinator 2 LGA NTD Officer 1 State NTD Officer	Ibadan North, Akinyele
5	Stakeholders in academia	3 Researchers	University of Ibadan

[1] The community in Akinyele did not have residential traditional healer or PMV.

2.4. Data Collection

We used a qualitative approach to data collection. Semi-structured interview guides with open-ended questions were developed based on the case management steps of schistosomiasis [15] and the health-seeking pathway in low-resource contexts [27] (See Figure 1). Van der Werf [15] describes the steps in passive case detection of schistosomiasis from a health care system perspective. She distinguishes five steps in the passive case detection as a liner process of infection, pathology, disease, health care visiting, and treatment. From practice and the literature, we are aware that the trajectory is more complex and can have multiple pathways within and outside the formal healthcare system. For example, informal health care providers such as Patent Medicine Vendors (PMVs) and traditional healers are known to be frequently the first choice of health-seeking by communities in Nigeria [28,29]. For this reason, we searched for a complementary model that would represent the complexity and alternative routes of healthcare-seeking behaviour of patients in Sub-Saharan Africa. This led to the work of R. E. Kohler et al. [27] who developed a six-stage health-seeking pathway based on interviews with women from Malawi. Even though their research was related to the early detection of breast cancer, it describes the complex trajectories of patients within the African context. We constructed a health-seeking pathway with six stages that was used to derive the main themes to be addressed. The questions were formulated to cover all the themes and to guide the semi-structured interviews (See Figure 1).

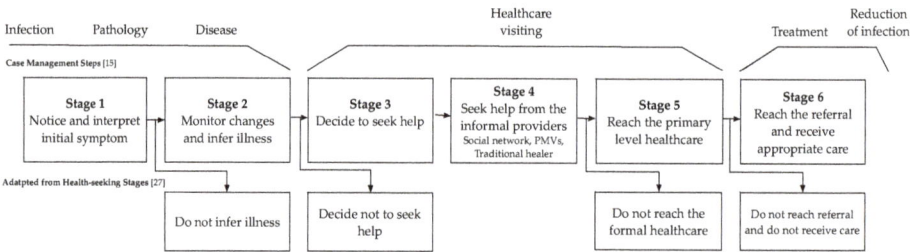

Figure 1. Adapted health-seeking pathway with six stages based on [15,27].

The study adopted a descriptive exploratory design using qualitative methods [Key informant Interview (KII) and In-depth Interview (IDI)]. The KIIs were conducted to explore the perspectives of the patients and health workers in accessing and performing the diagnosis and the case management, and IDIs to gain a broader understanding of challenges and collect insights for opportunities. The interviews were conducted in English or Yoruba (local language) for 45 min.

2.5. Data Entry and Analysis

All interviews were recorded and transcribed verbatim. Interviews conducted in Yoruba were translated into English by an external translator and reviewed by a language knowledge expert to ensure that the original meaning was not lost. Transcripts were analysed using the software Atlas ti version 8.4.4.

The framework of theory of access to healthcare was used to structure the data analysis and identify the barriers to access the case management of schistosomiasis. The 5A framework by Penchansky and Thomas's [30], which includes affordability, availability, accessibility, adequacy (or accommodation) and acceptability, is commonly used. However, we adopted Saurman's 6A Framework in our analysis because of an additional dimension on awareness considering its importance in remote and rural areas [31].

The lead researcher used pre-defined themes based on the 6A Framework on access to healthcare [31] to assign the codes using a deductive approach. The six analysed dimensions, described by their definitions and components adopted from another study [32] are shown in Table 2. Additionally, new themes were identified by inductive coding. The initial coding was done by the lead researcher and later reviewed by two other researchers of the team. This resulted in a list of barriers to access to schistosomiasis case management. Next, the themes and barriers were discussed and grouped into the six health seeking stages. Finally, the barriers were described based on (a) the six stages of the health seeking pathway and (b) in Figure 2; by the 6As of the health access framework using the health seeker or provider perspectives.

Table 2. 6A Framework of access to healthcare.

Dimensions	Component	Theme
Awareness	Communication and information	General health literacy Knowledge about symptoms, care and prevention
Accessibility	Location	Distribution of, and distance to, health care providers
Availability	Supply and demand	Incomplete medical infrastructure Lack of equipment Lack of health care professionals Lack of training for health care professionals
Acceptability	Consumer perception	Cultural belief and influence from the community
Affordability	Financial and incidental costs	Cost of treatment Cost of transport to health care provider
Adequacy (Accommodation)	Organisation	Mismatch between available information and awareness, knowledge, and education needs Lack of relevant and complete diagnostic information

3. Results

3.1. Health-Seeking Stages Identified in the Case Management

Based on the interviews, the six stages of the patient health-seeking pathway within the case management (See Figure 1) are described by common health-seeking behaviours. Next, identified themes within each stage which act as barriers are mentioned. The overview of the themes within 6A framework can be found in the table in Appendix A.

3.1.1. Stage 1: Notice and Interpret the Initial Symptoms

All the six 'category 1' interviewees mention the notification of blood in urine as an initial symptom for recognition of illness. Discomfort when urinating and fever were mentioned as well.

> *"I told her mum to keep her eyes on him, and she later saw him urinate and sighted blood in his urine, ... "*.
> —Parent of a child who had schistosomiasis from Rural LGA

In most cases described, identification of symptoms drew the immediate attention of the community members. However, lack of knowledge and other associations connected to the symptoms became barriers for community members to seek for health support (for schistosomiasis).

- Theme 1: Lack of general knowledge on health and schistosomiasis among community.

It was often mentioned that the general understanding within the community related to healthcare is low, which leads to less active attitudes in seeking care. More specifically, the community's knowledge of schistosomiasis related to the cause, signs, and symptoms of the disease were limited. This lack of knowledge makes it difficult for the community to interpret the symptoms, even though they noticed the initial signs.

- Theme 2: Cultural association and belief related to the symptoms

The symptoms are associated with cultural identity or beliefs within the community. This affects people not to seek for help and choose for traditional medicines in stage 4.

"I said it's like a cultural thing, once you have haematuria, that normalises you as a true son of the soil ... " —Public Health Researcher

"You know that dogs have blood in their urine. In the Southwest of Nigeria, it is called Atosi Aja. This is why they believe that it is not a medical condition and they prefer treating it traditionally" —PHC Coordinator (Rural LGA)

"Some people are aware of schistosomiasis, but most people believe that the spiritual forces have cursed the victim" —Community mobilizer (Urban LGA)

3.1.2. Stage 2: Monitor Changes and Infer Illness

After people become aware of the symptoms, they have the tendency to wait for several days before they take action. They monitor the symptoms and wait for the conditions to improve. It was mentioned by the guardians and parents of the patients that the symptoms are frequently associated with other diseases, for example, Sexually Transmitted Diseases (STDs). This makes people reluctant to seek care.

"after five days ... , okay you want to see if his condition will be better before deciding to take him to the hospital." —Parent of a child who had schistosomiasis (Rural LGA)

- Theme 3: Trying out self-medication without prescription

While monitoring the symptoms, it is common to make use of over-the-counter medications such as paracetamol or make traditional medicine at home. If the symptoms seem to disappear, people do not further seek for help. This reduces the chance of receiving appropriate care.

"We gave him paracetamol and yet there was no difference, he was sweating, and we took him outside to take fresh air ... " —Parent of a child who had schistosomiasis (Rural LGA)

3.1.3. Stage 3: Decide to Seek Help

Only after the symptom persists or becomes more severe do people decide to seek help. The patients consulted with their close ones in the community about their symptoms and where to seek help.

"Where I (people community) will go next is dependent on that. For instance, if I speak to a friend who is a pastor and he asks me to come to his church for healing prayers, then I would go to the church. If someone says that they had once experienced such and they saw a Community Health Extension Workers (CHEW), I would follow suit." —Doctor PHC (Urban LGA)

According to the level of knowledge in healthcare and socioeconomic status, the patients choose where to seek help in the next stage. In the community, people also preferred seeking help from the informal healthcare providers such as traditional healers and PMVs considering the accessibility and affordability (Stage 4). Depending on the relationship with health workers, sometimes they reach out the formal healthcare directly (Stage 5).

- Theme 4: The symptoms are associated with STD, which causes hesitation in sharing with others.

Due to the stigma around the STD, this type of misinterpretation causes unnecessary fear and confusion.

" ... it is possible that it is a sexually transmitted disease ... So it is possible that people may contract the disease but may be too shy or lack the courage to tell someone because of losing their dignity and privacy." —Guardian of child who had schistosomiasis (Urban LGA)

3.1.4. Stage 4: Seek Help from the Social Network and Informal Healthcare Providers

Stage 4.1. Seeking Help from Social Network

It is common to start seeking help by consulting other community members and ask for advice from someone who had similar experiences. Patients discuss with a trusted person such as family, friends, or other community members.

> *"He said it just found out he urinated blood . . . . so when he mentioned it was where his apprentice told him there is someone that treated him when he contracted the same disease . . . "* —Traditional healer (Urban LGA)

> *" . . . he confided in someone that he had contracted the disease and I got to know through that person though I was warned not to ask him or pretend as if I am not aware . . . "* —Guardian of a child who had schistosomiasis (Urban LGA)

- Theme 5: Limited access to the proper information within the community due to low awareness on schistosomiasis

Since there is generally little knowledge on Schistosomiasis, it is difficult for patients to get access to the right information via their social network.

> *"he has never heard of it (schistosomiasis), he only knows about reddish urine . . . "* —Guardian of a child who had schistosomiasis 2 (Urban LGA)

Stage 4.2. Seeking Help through Traditional Medicine

Traditional medicine was believed as an effective solution, especially when other people had positive experiences to relieve the similar symptoms. Moreover, traditional healers are more accessible and affordable as they are easily approached from the community, and the cost of treatment is relatively low. The belief that the disease is related to spiritual power (Theme 2) also influences patients to choose the traditional healers, who are respected among the community.

> *"they probably just tell them "oh it is spiritual problem" "Oh, it's not normal, it's something spiritual..."* —Public Health Researcher

> *"It depends on customs and traditions. It also depends on the condition because they may think that the disease is as a result of witchcraft and wizardry..."* —PHC Coordinator (Rural LGA)

Stage 4.3. Seeking Over-the-Counter Medications from PMVs or Drug Vendors

Purchasing medicines from the PMVs or drug vendors were mentioned as a typical behaviour for health-seeking. Especially in rural communities, people prefer to buy over-the-counter medicines such as paracetamol and try self-medication as described in Theme 3. The patients or the guardians visit the PMVs and consult symptoms or ask for a specific medicine. For previous cases of schistosomiasis, they purchased antibiotics and paracetamol without prescription. The health workers referred to this process as trial-and-error where patients trying out the given medicines for one to three days and come back if not effective. If the conditions of the patients are too serious for the PMVs to handle, the PMVs provide a referral for the patients to visit the health centre.

> *"I usually bought drugs from drug vendors that hawks . . . "* —Mother with a treated child with schistosomiasis (Rural LGA)

> *"They want immediate solutions, so they first buy herbs or patronize the PMVs."* —Community Mobilizer/CHO (Rural LGA)

"Because of ignorance, the people go to them because they are at every nook and cranny" —MOH/PHC Coordinator (Urban LGA)

- Theme 6: Going through the process of trial-and-error medications without prescriptions at the PMVs.

Taking medicines without a prescription is not only causing a delay in receiving the proper care but also develops resistance to drugs such as antibiotics.

"They mostly do trial and error just in a bid to make money regardless of lacking knowledge … " —NTD Officer (Urban LGA)

3.1.5. Stage 5: Reach the Primary Level Healthcare

The CHEWs or health workers at primary health centre provide health-related education on common diseases and build a close relationship with the community. This relationship increases the chance of community members contacting them or health centre when they become ill. The four community health workers we interviewed reportedly had a strong relationship with community members which positively influenced the patients' health-seeking pathway.

"The PHC is a bit far away from their places but they still come around because of the relationship we have with them." —CHEW (Rural LGA)

Considering the misinterpretation of the symptoms (Theme 4), the trust between the patients and a health worker is important to open up about the symptoms.

"Based on the relationship we have with them; they can easily tell us without feeling embarrassed or shy … . They know me, and I have been with them for a long time." —Community mobilizer (Rural LGA)

- Theme 7: Negative attitudes of the health workers may prevent people from accessing formal health care.

The negative attitudes of some of the health workers may become potential barriers to access formal health care.

"The attitude needs to be improved so that we can be more receptive to these people" —MOH/PHC Coordinator (Urban LGA)

"We make sure things are friendly and simplified in order to make sure they are not scared … " —NTD Officer (Urban LGA)

Stage 5.1. Consultation

The consultation with health workers starts from asking about the symptoms and the patient history. If schistosomiasis is suspected, possible contact with water is also asked. The time to get attended was not considered as a challenge in both LGAs.

"When the patients are brought to the clinic, we ask about the complaints, we find out if the child bathes near wells and rivers and they say yes...." —Community mobilizer (Rural LGA)

Once the health care workers recognize the symptoms and suspect schistosomiasis, there are two actions they should take. First, provide the appropriate case management or refer the patients to another health centre or hospital where the patients can receive the care.

Secondly, report to the Local Government as schistosomiasis to be included in the Integrated Disease Surveillance Response program. This will call the attention of the Disease Surveillance Notification Officer (DSNO), and the DSNO who will initiate the surveillance protocol to collect a sample and confirm the case. For the surveillance protocol, the DSNO collects the sample and brings it to a qualified laboratory for diagnosis. However, this does not take place for unreported cases.

- Theme 8: Knowledge gap of high-risk groups of schistosomiasis among the community

The stakeholders at the community level (Categories 2, 3) often mentioned that the prevalence is low in the LGAs where the interviews took place. However, the higher-level stakeholders (Categories 4, 5) mentioned specific communities are at higher risk of schistosomiasis, for example, around the riverine areas, which is not recognized by the health workers and cause low awareness. This is a clear gap in knowledge that can lead to the cases being missed and underreported.

> "In Ibadan (city), for instance, there is a location called Dandaaru. It is around University College Hospital. People live around that community and their children go there to bath. In the process, they get infected with schistosomiasis." —Public health researcher

- Theme 9: Failure in suspecting the case based on symptoms

Most health workers are familiar with blood in urine, but they may not associate the symptoms with schistosomiasis case. In addition, there may be non-specific symptoms which makes it difficult for the health workers to identify the case. This prevents the patients from receiving the appropriate care for schistosomiasis, and the surveillance program will miss the case.

> "if a patient comes with a case of blood in their urine and if the health worker does not have adequate knowledge to say that it is similar to schistosomiasis, there is no way the patient can take a step further to investigate ... There may be misdiagnosis and some cases may be entirely missed. Some may have the disease and assume that it is a sexually transmitted infections ... Training of the health workers to build their skills to detect schistosomiasis is very important." —MOH/PHC Coordinator (Urban LGA)

> "I'm not sure maybe 5 or 9 of them had a microscopic (haematuria) and not the haematuria ... it wasn't like they came with symptoms." —Public health researcher

Stage 5.2. Diagnosis

Once a schistosomiasis case is suspected, a diagnosis should take place to confirm the case and provide treatment. Preventing wastage of free medication from the health centres is another factor mentioned.

> "You must carry out urinalysis with at least simple microscopy. It is very important to know what you are dealing with and to rule out certain thing ... " —MOH/PHC (Urban LGA)

> "Diagnosis is very important because, without it, no treatment can be made." —PHC Coordinator (Rural LGA)

The diagnosis will be performed within the facility if a laboratory is available and functioning. We inquired the lab scientists about the standard method for schistosomiasis which was confirmed as urine analysis. It involves the collection of a urine sample, sample preparation, urine strip tests, and microscopic analysis. Urine filtration was not mentioned by any of the four labs we visited. The sample preparation was done by centrifuge as a standard procedure.

> "Now a patient comes to the laboratory and the physician has requested a urinalysis, for a urine analysis and a urine microscopy" —Lab scientist (Urban LGA)

However, none of the four health centres we visited had a functioning laboratory in place. The barriers include incomplete infrastructure and lack of equipment, unstable electricity and power supply, and lack of qualified health care professionals.

- Theme 10: Incomplete medical infrastructure to perform diagnosis

In the primary health centre, there was a lack of adequate equipment to perform the microscopy such as centrifuge, microscope, clean and controlled environment, and a stable supply of electricity. The size of the space and the environment (excessive heat, exposure to sunlight) were also mentioned as reasons why the facility was not functioning.

"There is no machine (microscope). We do have labs, but we are limited to some tests to be carried out at the LGA level." —NTD Officer (Rural LGA)

"But at times, when we don't have equipment, we call our boss and ask to either to refer the patient or if he is on his way down, if he is, he would bring the equipment needed from Moniya by his bike … " —CHEW (Rural LGA)

Unstable power supply was another factor due to which microscopy cannot function properly. As an alternative solution, the generator was mentioned, but only two of the visited labs were equipped with it. The generators were functioning at the moment, but it was also mentioned that the generators frequently break down and do not function. Maintenance of the broken devices was an additional challenge especially when they do not have a back-up device.

"there is currently no power supply. We have an old generator and there is no money … " —Lab scientist (Urban LGA)

- Theme 11: Lack of lab scientists and technicians to perform diagnosis

The absence of lab scientists was a recurring issue at the primary level health centres. Among the four labs we visited, we interviewed at least one lab scientists or technician. In two labs attached to the primary health centre, only lab technicians were present. Even if they are available, potential insufficient training of the professionals was considered as a barrier.

" … Then manpower should be on ground. Scientists, more scientists should be on ground so that the work won't be too much on individuals … " —Lab scientist at PHC (Urban LGA)

"She is a laboratory technician, not a full scientist. She is just a technician … " When asked about the lab personnel at the PHC– Head of PHC (Urban LGA)

- Theme 12: Incapability to perform the diagnosis with sufficient quality

One academic stakeholder mentioned that the lack of skills of lab scientists and technicians is one of the challenging factors to deliver diagnostic results with sufficient quality.

"the skill of their laboratory technician is not good enough to pick that, then you might miss even if there are 100 cases in that community … " —Public Health Researcher

- Theme 13: Extra steps of movements are required for diagnosis and treatment.
- Theme 14: The costs incurred for extra steps are patient's responsibilities.

At the health centre without diagnostic capacity, diagnosis may be requested from other facilities. In this case, it is the responsibility of the patient to reach there and bring the results back for treatment. Some patients may not continue the health-seeking pathways due to the extra costs of transportation and time incurred. It was mentioned that the costs of diagnosis and treatment are free at the health centre. However, if these are not available at the health centre, it is under patients' own expenses to go to a private lab for diagnosis or pharmacy for treatment.

"our people are still poor, if test is expensive they will say they will come back … . She told me she didn't have enough money on her for the test that she had only five hundred naira … " —Guardian of child who had schistosomiasis II (Urban LGA)

Stage 5.3. Symptom-Based Diagnosis and Treatment

In prior cases of schistosomiasis, health workers have provided treatment based on symptoms without diagnosis. The lack of knowledge of the health workers not only caused schistosomiasis case to be missed, but also questioned the reliability of the symptom-based treatment.

"We combine the signs and symptoms with the patient history of the patient . . . We treated them clinically as we did not have any laboratory to confirm it." —Community Mobilizer (Rural LGA)

- Theme 15: The symptom-based treatments are not always reliable.

The stakeholders from category 4 and 6 mentioned that the symptom-based treatment is not always reliable. As mentioned in theme 8 and 9, the case may not be suspected at all or fall under misdiagnosis or mistreatment.

"Even on clinical level, such a diagnosis can be missed . . . So, when you have this patient and you do not use your initiative to conclude that you have to conduct urinalysis with microscopy on this patient, it is possible to miss the diagnosis . . . " —MOH/PHC Coordinator (Urban LGA)

Stage 5.4. Treatment and Follow-Up

Generally, the treatment will be provided according to the results of the diagnosis. In the previous cases, the treatment was given before receiving the diagnostic results. Even when DSNO requested the diagnosis, the treatment was given without waiting for confirmation due to the delay in receiving the results.

- Theme 16: Treatment is given before the test results are available.

This happened when there was a delay in receiving the results. For the convenience of the patients, the treatment was given immediately, so they do not have to come back for the results and treatment—This relates back to the barriers in accessibility and affordability.

"After everything, my boss told me they got drugs and that it was schistosomiasis. However, I did not see the laboratory results." —CHEW (Rural LGA)

"If you ask the patient to go home without giving them anything, they will not come back to you. This is why you have to reassure and give them something without the case being confirmed" —PHC Coordinator (Rural LGA)

The follow-up takes place by the health workers to check on recovery via personal contact or phone call.

"after that they will tell them to take their drugs properly, they will also tell them to do check-up either the following or after two days . . . " —Guardian of a child who had schistosomiasis II (Urban LGA)

3.1.6. Stage 6: Reach the Referral and Receive Appropriate Care

From the primary health care, the patients are referred to visit an advanced level of health care facility. In the areas we conducted our study, the Hospital affiliated to the University of Ibadan was often mentioned as a referral and, in most cases, patients followed the advice for schistosomiasis and other diseases. Once they reach the referral hospital, the patients received the appropriate care with diagnosis and treatment. However, there were still barriers such as the long-distance to the healthcare provider, the transportation costs and the general fear of health care.

- Theme 17: Distance to the health care provider is far.
- Theme 18: Transportation costs are unaffordable.

In the communities located in urban areas, access to the referred healthcare facility such as hospital was not described as a challenge. However, in the rural communities, the distance to the healthcare facility was major challenge in access as well as costs of transportation. Moreover, it was described that the patients might have to depend on other family members or neighbours to arrange transportation which cause additional delay in seeking care. One health worker mentioned that she offers to provide the transportation costs when she gives a referral. The time to travel to the health care provider was also seen as a challenge.

"Even transportation is a cause for concern. They want immediate attention and asking them to go to another hospital is like adding salt to their journey . . . " —Community mobilizer/CHO (Rural LGA)

"Even if free drugs are available at the hospital, they have to think of the transport fare from their house to the hospital." —PHC Coordinator (Rural LGA)

- Theme 19: Fear of healthcare facility and uncertainty make people hesitant to reach referral

Another barrier identified was the general fear for healthcare facility as the hospital was usually associated with a place "with stress" due to their prior experiences. The fear comes from the uncertainty of the further process in which they might have to spend excessive time and costs.

"We have heard of cases of people with phobias for health center that close their eyes when they walk pass by the facility" —NTD officer (Urban LGA)

"I said fear and shyness, fear that they will be admitted (to hospital) and may not be allowed to come go back home . . . " —Guardian of child who had schistosomiasis (Urban LGA)

3.2. Barriers to the Case Management and Diagnosis

In the final stage, the identified barriers were grouped according to the six stages of the healthcare seeking pathway and the 6A dimensions of access to healthcare (See Figure 2). It is also indicated if the barriers were from the perspectives of healthcare seeker or a provider.

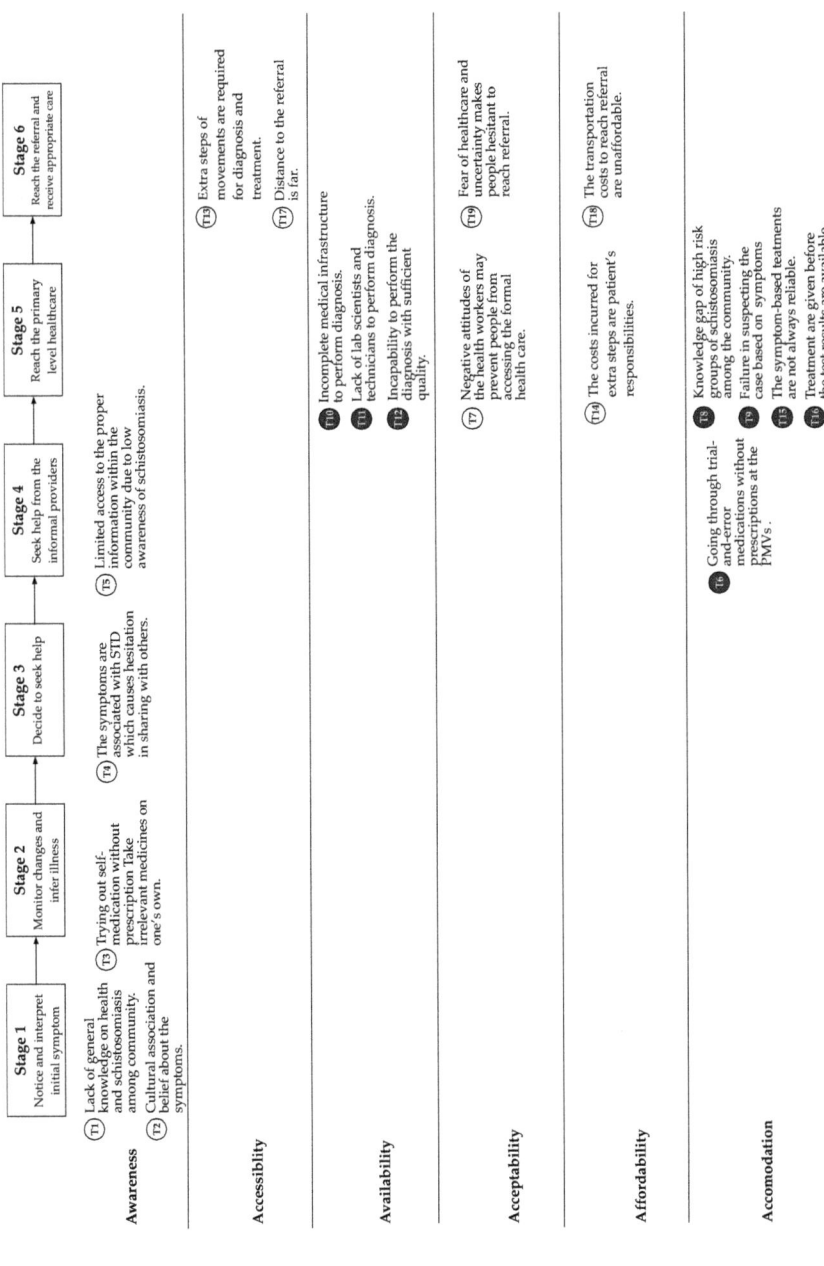

Figure 2. Identified barriers in the case management and diagnosis in 6A Framework. ○ = Barriers from the healthcare seeker perspectives, ● = Barriers from the healthcare provider perspectives.

4. Discussion

4.1. Main Findings

This study explored the health-seeking behaviours of patients and the diagnostic capability of the primary healthcare level in schistosomiasis case management in Oyo State, Nigeria. Based on the results, we identified barriers to access to adequate health care and diagnosis. The overall health-seeking pathway was found to be in line with the pathway as identified in the literature [15,27]. We elaborated on the health-seeking behaviours and barriers within each stage specifically related to schistosomiasis. Overall, the barriers from the healthcare seeker perspectives were spread over all six stages (See Appendix A). The disease awareness was major barrier for the patients at the beginning of the health-seeking pathway, followed by accessibility and affordability. The barriers from the provider perspectives were more present in the later stage of pathway (Stage 5 and 6) where the availability of diagnostics and disease detection rates by the health worker were challenging factors. During the interview, no other categories of health-seeking stages and barriers to access were mentioned which indicates the validity of the framework we used.

As mentioned in previous studies [24,25], awareness was one of the main barriers. Within our empirical study, a lack of awareness was spread over several stages of the health-seeking pathway. The barriers to awareness are more present in the early stages of health-seeking before visiting the health facilities and from the patients' perspectives. The low awareness of the disease and other associations connected to the symptoms in the community resulted in delay in seeking healthcare and self-medication. The patients often choose alternative routes (PMVs and traditional medicine) before they reach formal healthcare. This is similar to the health-seeking behaviour of other common diseases [28,29] using trial and errors of medication without prescription which causes delay in accessing care.

When patients seek out formal health care, schistosomiasis is often underestimated by the health workers. The barriers to the acceptability strongly influenced the decision-making where the health care workers attitudes and perception of formal health care were the major issues. The health care providers have multiple barriers related to accommodation including the knowledge gap and non-specific symptoms of the disease. Even when the case is suspected, the health care providers face challenges in providing laboratory confirmation of the case due to unavailability of the diagnostic equipment and personnel. The unavailability issues were directly related to the incomplete infrastructure, lack of training of personnel, and environmental challenges such as power supply. This leads to failure in following the recommended procedure of the case management and raises additional barriers to accommodation. The symptom-based treatment, which is alternative to diagnosis, was found to be frequently not reliable due to the limited knowledge of the healthcare providers. Referral to another diagnostic facility is possible but the delay in receiving the result led to treating the patients without confirmation for the sake of convenience. Lastly, the referral to other facilities brings more burden of time and costs for the patients, which relates to the issues of accessibility and affordability.

4.2. Opportunities

Based on the identified barriers and comparing our findings with existing knowledge, we suggest following opportunities to improve access to the proper case management and diagnosis.

4.2.1. Community Sensitization Program for Awareness Creation

Active involvement of the community members for sensitization and health education will improve the general awareness on schistosomiasis by overcoming mis-associations around the symptoms and the passive attitudes in health-seeking behaviours. There is a need for focusing on the information on the disease causation, risk practices, key symptoms, consequences of the disease and delayed treatment. This will influence the community members to take desirable actions for prevention and seeking care once they notice early signs of the schistosomiasis. Multiple methods of dissemination should be used including informal healthcare providers such as traditional healers and PMVs.

4.2.2. A Study to Identify Prevalence of Schistosomiasis Among other High-Risk Groups

There is a need for a prevalence study focusing on other high-risk groups including the adults who frequently interact with water. Since children are already covered by the control and elimination program, this will help the health workers to realize the hidden burden of schistosomiasis in their local context. As the prevalence of schistosomiasis is perceived as low without evidence, schistosomiasis is "neglected" among the community and health workers. Presenting data specific to their local context will provide the health workers with awareness of the severity and urgency and consequently improve accommodation by providing the appropriate care for schistosomiasis. The prevalence study will generate needed evidence and guide the development of appropriate strategies for effective implementation of case management.

4.2.3. Enhancing the Existing Diagnostics Capacity

Stimulating adequate case management of schistosomiasis infection requires minimizing the number of steps by patients to reach the health centres where they can receive appropriate care. In this study, poor accessibility is evident with a concomitant effect on PHC utilisation. The issue of transportation costs due to referrals cannot be resolved without improving the accessibility and availability of the health workers and equipment. Enhancing the existing diagnostic capacity at the primary level will reduce the additional movements to reach other health facility and laboratories. Complementing the existing laboratory infrastructure, provided with more equipment and skilled personnel, will be necessary as well as providing solutions for other environmental factors such as unstable power supply.

4.2.4. Implementation of Point-of-Care Diagnostics Solution

Implementing an affordable and simple point-of-care diagnostics solution will reduce the financial burden of equipment and personnel at each health facility. Point-of-diagnostics can confirm the detected cases immediately and will reduce the risk of missed or misdiagnosed cases. It will be a favourable solution to allow the task distribution with minimal training, for example, by enabling community-based diagnosis by the community health workers. If the sensitivity is sufficient enough, the point-of-care diagnostics solution can be utilized for other opportunities such as prevalence study or community-based screening with higher affordability and accessibility. From the patient perspectives, additional travel and costs to the diagnostic facility are no longer necessary and there will be no delay in the results.

4.2.5. Community-Based Screening for Treatment and Monitoring

It would be a feasible approach to improve the availability of diagnostics at the primary healthcare level by adding schistosomiasis screening to other health care interventions already in place. This will likely have an immediate impact in reducing the number of infections and help in the collection of data for prevalence monitoring. A new diagnostic method available at the point-of-care with smart, high sensitivity and immediate output generation will add immense value to carry out such screening and would stimulate demand for services. This will be an advantage for the health centre in rural areas by preventing additional travel to the diagnostic facility.

4.2.6. Capability Strengthening of the Health Workers

Increasing the capability of the health workers will be a key to improve detection rate at the community level. More suitable approaches for different endemic levels should be determined based on the prevalence study and guide the health workers. The training of the health workers should include suspecting schistosomiasis cases from the symptoms and the contextual factors and emphasize the importance of the diagnostics. The availability of smart diagnostics will be beneficial to detect light infections or asymptomatic cases and avoid misdiagnosis. The willingness of people to seek help in formal health care was strongly influenced by the close relationship between the health workers and the community. Accordingly, the positive attitudes of the health workers towards the community should be emphasized in the training. New interventions should consider training the health care providers at the community level and the informal sector (PMVs and traditional medicine) to enhance collaboration between them. This will improve the awareness in the community.

4.3. Limitations of the Study

The limitations of this study should be noted. First, the patient's experience of schistosomiasis (stakeholder category 1) have taken place in the last 3 years. However, we were able to validate the findings and gain a more comprehensive understanding of other contextual and organizational factors through interviewing the multiple levels of stakeholders. The stories of the cases in the past were validated by confirming the facts with the health workers who put us in contact with the respondents as they were involved in the case as well. Second, the number of stakeholders were limited and they were selected from two LGAs, which can limit the generalizability of the results. Even though there was still limited access to health care and diagnostics, the LGAs were still considered to be close to the urban area (capital of the state). More studies can be conducted in more rural areas to deepen the understanding of barriers more specific to that context. Nevertheless, we believe the key findings and the identified barriers from this study are generalizable to similar settings and can be used to improve the case management of schistosomiasis.

Author Contributions: Conceptualization, methodology, first analysis and validation; G.-Y.V., A.O. and J.C.D.; software, G.-Y.V.; original draft preparation, G.-Y.V.; writing—review and editing, G.-Y.V., A.O., J.C.D., J.v.E. and O.O.; visualization, G.-Y.V.; supervision, J.C.D., J.v.E. and O.O.; project administration in the field study, O.O.; All authors have read and agreed to the published version of the manuscript.

Funding: Part of the research described has been funded by NWO-WOTRO Science for Global Develoment programme, grant number W 07.30318.009.

Acknowledgments: We thank Delft Global Initiative and our collaborators within the INSPiRED project who provided valuable support. We also thank Temitope Agbana for his support and encouragement. Special thanks to Opeyemi Oladunni for assistance in coordinating the field research and Merlijn Sluiter for her contribution in the interviews. We thank all the respondents who participated in our study, and a translator Yekinni Fatimat Oyinloluwa.

Conflicts of Interest: The funders had no role in the design of the study; in the collection, analyses, or interpretation of data; in the writing of the manuscript, or in the decision to publish the results.

Appendix A

Table A1. Barriers categorized in 6A dimensions and the perspectives.

6A Dimension	Barriers Identified	HC Seeker	HC Provider
Awareness	T1: Lack of general knowledge on health and schistosomiasis among community (Stage 1)	✓ [1]	
	T2: Cultural association and belief about the symptoms (Stage 1)	✓	
	T3: Trying out self-medication without prescription Take irrelevant medicines on one's own (Stage 2)	✓	
	T4: The symptoms are associated with STD which causes hesitation in sharing with others (Stage 3)	✓	
	T5: Limited access to the right information within the community due to low awareness of schistosomiasis (Stage 4)	✓	
Accessibility	T13: Extra steps of movements are required for diagnosis and treatment.	✓	
	T17: Distance to the referral is far (Stage 6)	✓	
Availability	T10: Incomplete medical infrastructure to perform diagnosis (Stage 5)		✓
	T11: Lack of lab scientists and technicians to perform diagnosis (Stage 5)		✓
	T12: Incapability to perform the diagnosis with sufficient quality (Stage 5)		✓

Table A1. *Cont.*

6A Dimension	Barriers Identified	HC Seeker	HC Provider
Acceptability	T7: Negative attitudes of the health workers may prevent people from accessing the formal health care (Stage 4)	√	
	T19: Fear of healthcare and uncertainty makes people hesitant to reach referral (Stage 5)	√	
Affordability	T14: The costs incurred for extra steps are patient's responsibilities.	√	
	T18: The transportation costs to reach referral are unaffordable (Stage 6)	√	
Adequacy/ Accommodation	T6: Going through trial-and-error medications without prescriptions at the PMVs (Stage 4)		√
	T8: Knowledge gap of high risk groups of schistosomiasis among the community (Stage 5)		√
	T9: Failure in suspecting the case based on symptoms (Stage 5)		√
	T15: The symptom-based treatments are not always available (Stage 5)		√
	T18: Treatment are given before the test results are available. (Stage 5)		√

[1] Checkmark √ indicates from which perspective the barrier is found.

References

1. Savioli, L.; Engels, D.; Roungou, J.B.; Fenwick, A.; Endo, H. Schistosomiasis control. *Lancet* **2004**, *20*, 363–658. [CrossRef]
2. Ezeh, C.O.; Onyekwelu, K.C.; Akinwale, O.P.; Shan, L.; Wei, H. Urinary schistosomiasis in Nigeria: A 50 year review of prevalence, distribution and disease burden. *Parasite* **2019**, *26*, 19. [CrossRef] [PubMed]
3. King, C.H. Parasites and poverty: The case of schistosomiasis. *Acta Trop.* **2010**, *113*, 95–104. [CrossRef] [PubMed]
4. Adenowo, A.F.; Oyinloye, B.E.; Ogunyinka, B.I.; Kappo, A.P. Impact of human schistosomiasis in sub-Saharan Africa. *Braz. J. Infect. Dis.* **2015**, *19*, 196–205. [CrossRef]
5. Federal Ministry of Health. Report on Epidemiological Mapping of Schistosomiasis and Soil Transmitted Helminthiasis in 19 States and the FCT, Nigeria. 2015. Available online: www.health.gov.ng/doc/SchistoSTH.pdf (accessed on 1 April 2020).
6. Mafe, M.A.; Von Stamm, T.; Utzinger, J.; N'goran, E.K. Control of urinary schistosomiasis: An investigation into the effective use of questionnaires to identify high-risk communities and individuals in Niger State, Nigeria. *Trop. Med. Int. Health* **2000**, *5*, 53–63. [CrossRef]
7. Evans, D.S.; King, J.D.; Eigege, A.; Umaru, J.; Adamani, W.; Alphonsus, K.; Sambo, Y.; Miri, E.S.; Goshit, D.; Ogah, G.; et al. Assessing the WHO 50% prevalence threshold in school-aged children as indication for treatment of urogenital schistosomiasis in adults in central Nigeria. *Am. J. Trop. Med. Hyg.* **2013**, *88*, 441–445. [CrossRef]
8. Mafe, M.A.; Appelt, B.; Adewale, B.; Idowu, E.T.; Akinwale, O.P.; Adeneye, A.K.; Manafa, O.U.; Sulyman, M.A.; Akande, O.D.; Omotola, B.D. Effectiveness of different approaches to mass delivery of praziquantel among school-aged children in rural communities in Nigeria. *Acta Trop.* **2005**, *93*, 181–190. [CrossRef]
9. Bruun, B.; Aagaard-Hansen, J. *The Social Context of Schistosomiasis and Its Control*; World Health Organisation: Geneva, Switzerland, 2008; pp. 118–119.
10. Hopkins, D.R.; Eigege, A.; Miri, E.S.; Gontor, I.; Ogah, G.; Umaru, J.; Gwomkudu, C.C.; Mathai, W.; Jinadu, M.Y.; Amadiegwu, S.; et al. Lymphatic filariasis elimination and schistosomiasis control in combination with onchocerciasis control in Nigeria. *Am. J. Trop. Med. Hyg.* **2002**, *67*, 266–272. [CrossRef]
11. Richards, F.O., Jr.; Eigege, A.; Miri, E.S.; Jinadu, M.Y.; Hopkins, D.R. Integration of mass drug administration programmes in Nigeria: The challenge of schistosomiasis. *Bull. World Health Organ.* **2006**, *84*, 673–676. [CrossRef]
12. N'Goran, E.K.; Utzinger, J.; N'guessan, A.N.; Müller, I.; Zamblé, K.; Lohourignon, K.L.; Traoré, M.; Sosthène, B.A.; Lengeler, C.; Tanner, M. Reinfection with *Schistosoma haematobium* following school-based chemotherapy with praziquantel in four highly endemic villages in Côte d'Ivoire. *Trop. Med. Int. Health* **2001**, *6*, 817–825. [CrossRef]
13. Utzinger, J.; Raso, G.; Brooker, S.; De Savigny, D.; Tanner, M.; Ørnbjerg, N.; Singer, B.H.; N'goran, E.K. Schistosomiasis and neglected tropical diseases: Towards integrated and sustainable control and a word of caution. *Parasitology* **2009**, *136*, 1859–1874. [CrossRef] [PubMed]

14. Chiamah, O.C.; Ubachukwu, P.O.; Anorue, C.O.; Ebi, S. Urinary schistosomiasis in Ebonyi State, Nigeria from 2006 to 2017. *J. Vector Borne Dis.* **2019**, *56*, 87–91. [CrossRef] [PubMed]
15. van der Werf, M. Schistosomiasis Morbidity and Management of Cases in Africa. Ph.D. Thesis, Erasmus University Rotterdam, Rotterdam, The Netherlands, 21 May 2003.
16. World Health Organisation. *The Control of Schistosomiasis*; Technical Report Series; No. 728; World Health Organisation: Geneva, Switzerland, 1993.
17. Utzinger, J.; Becker, S.L.; Van Lieshout, L.; Van Dam, G.J.; Knopp, S. New diagnostic tools in schistosomiasis. *Clin. Microbiol. Infect.* **2015**, *21*, 529–542. [CrossRef]
18. Ajibola, O.; Gulumbe, B.H.; Eze, A.A.; Obishakin, E. Tools for detection of schistosomiasis in resource limited settings. *Med. Sci.* **2018**, *6*, 39. [CrossRef] [PubMed]
19. Urdea, M.; Penny, L.A.; Olmsted, S.S.; Giovanni, M.Y.; Kaspar, P.; Shepherd, A.; Wilson, P.; Dahl, C.A.; Buchsbaum, S.; Moeller, G.; et al. Requirements for high impact diagnostics in the developing world. *Nature* **2006**, *444*, 73–79. [CrossRef] [PubMed]
20. De Vlas, S.J.; Danso-Appiah, A.; Van Der Werf, M.J.; Bosompem, K.M.; Habbema, J.D.F. Quantitative evaluation of integrated schistosomiasis control: The example of passive case finding in Ghana. *Trop. Med. Int. Health* **2004**, *9*, A16–A21. [CrossRef] [PubMed]
21. van der Werf, M.J.; de Vlas, S.J.; Landouré, A.; Bosompem, K.M.; Habbema, J.D.F. Measuring schistosomiasis case management of the health services in Ghana and Mali. *Trop. Med. Int. Health* **2004**, *9*, 149–157. [CrossRef]
22. Oyekale, A.S. Assessment of primary health care facilities' service readiness in Nigeria. *BMC Health Serv. Res.* **2017**, *17*, 172. [CrossRef]
23. Ehiri, J.E.; Oyo-Ita, A.E.; Anyanwu, E.C.; Meremikwu, M.M.; Ikpeme, M.B. Quality of child health services in primary health care facilities in south-east Nigeria. *Child Care Health Dev.* **2005**, *31*, 181–191. [CrossRef]
24. Dawaki, S.; Al-Mekhlafi, H.M.; Ithoi, I.; Ibrahim, J.; Abdulsalam, A.M.; Ahmed, A.; Sady, H.; Nasr, N.A.; Atroosh, W.M. The menace of schistosomiasis in Nigeria: Knowledge, attitude, and practices regarding schistosomiasis among rural communities in Kano State. *PLoS ONE* **2015**, *10*, e0143667. [CrossRef]
25. Tidi, S.K.; Jummai, A.T. Urinary schistosomiasis: Health seeking behaviour among residents of Kiri in Shelleng Local Government Area of Adamawa state. *J. Environ. Toxicol. Publ. Health* **2015**, *1*, 30–35.
26. National Bureau of Statistics. *2017, Demographic Statistics Bulletin*; National Bureau of Statistics: Abuja, Nigeria, 2018; p. 8.
27. Kohler, R.E.; Gopal, S.; Miller, A.R.; Lee, C.N.; Reeve, B.B.; Weiner, B.J.; Wheeler, S.B. A framework for improving early detection of breast cancer in sub-Saharan Africa: A qualitative study of help-seeking behaviors among Malawian women. *Patient Educ. Couns.* **2017**, *100*, 167–173. [CrossRef] [PubMed]
28. Oladepo, O.; Salami, K.K.; Adeoye, B.W.; Oshiname, F.; Ofi, B.; Oladepo, M.; Ogunbemi, O.; Lawal, A.; Brieger, W.R.; Bloom, G.; et al. *Malaria Treatment and Policy in Three Regions in Nigeria: The Role of Patent Medicine Vendors*; Future Health Systems, 2007; pp. 1–29.
29. Bloom, G.; Standing, H.; Lucas, H.; Bhuiya, A.; Oladepo, O.; Peters, D.H. Making health markets work better for poor people: The case of informal providers. *Health Policy Plan.* **2011**, *26* (Suppl. 1), i45–i52. [CrossRef] [PubMed]
30. Saurman, E. Improving access: Modifying Penchansky and Thomas's theory of access. *J. Health Serv. Res. Policy* **2016**, *21*, 36–39. [CrossRef]
31. Penchansky, R.; Thomas, J.W. The concept of access: Definition and relationship to consumer satisfaction. *Med. Care* **1981**, *19*, 127–140. [CrossRef]
32. Iwamoto, R.; Santos, A.L.R.; Chavannes, N.; Reis, R.; Diehl, J.C. Considerations for an Access-Centered Design of the Fever Thermometer in Low-Resource Settings: A Literature Review. *JMIR Hum. Factors* **2017**, *4*, e3. [CrossRef]

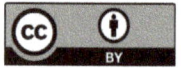

© 2020 by the authors. Licensee MDPI, Basel, Switzerland. This article is an open access article distributed under the terms and conditions of the Creative Commons Attribution (CC BY) license (http://creativecommons.org/licenses/by/4.0/).

MDPI
St. Alban-Anlage 66
4052 Basel
Switzerland
Tel. +41 61 683 77 34
Fax +41 61 302 89 18
www.mdpi.com

Diagnostics Editorial Office
E-mail: diagnostics@mdpi.com
www.mdpi.com/journal/diagnostics

www.ingramcontent.com/pod-product-compliance
Lightning Source LLC
LaVergne TN
LVHW070615100526
838202LV00012B/651